Essential Revision Notes for the FRCS (Urol)

2nd edition

Jack Donati-Bourne

Volume 2

Foreword by
Keith Yeates Gold Medal Winners
Rachel Barratt and Sotonye Tolofari

First published in 2025 by Libri Publishing

ISBN 978-1-911451-37-2

Cover and Design by Carnegie Publishing

Libri Publishing
Brunel House
Volunteer Way
Faringdon
Oxfordshire
SN7 7YR

Tel: +44 (0)845 873 3837

www.libripublishing.co.uk

CONTENTS

DEDICATION

This book is dedicated to Zakariya, my beautiful precious boy.

ABOUT THE AUTHOR

Jack Donati-Bourne works as a Consultant Urological Surgeon in Sandwell and West Birmingham Hospitals NHS Trust. He qualified in medicine (2010) and then obtained a Master's degree in anatomy (2013), both at the University of Birmingham, proceeding subsequently to complete Membership (2013) and Fellowship (2019) of the Royal College of Surgeons of England.

He has published 20 articles in peer-reviewed journals and his work has been presented in eight different countries. The first edition of the *Essential Revision Notes for the FRCS (Urol)* textbook was sold across the world.

Jack has a passion for the NHS and teaching, aiming to support and inspire trainees along the way, which was the driving force behind the production of the textbooks.

FOREWORD

I had sat through three years of high-class urology teaching and yet, as I approached my exam year, I realised I had no clue where or how to start my revision for the FRCS (Urol) exam. I started making notes – scraping information from any source I could find – followed by a mad month of cramming at the end. Sadly, I sat my FRCS (Urol) at the same time as Jack Donati-Bourne and didn't have the fortune to have a textbook that gave me such a solid foundation from which to start my revision. So, congratulations – if you are reading this then you are already a step ahead. Whilst I also advise writing additional notes yourself, this book will allow you to really focus your time on assimilating and understanding the information.

Revision for Part 1 is, to put it mildly, dull, lonely and life consuming. Everyone has their own way of revising for written exams. I spent three months writing notes (a job this book makes easier for you!) with a revision timetable roughly split to give more time to larger topics and less to shorter topics or those with which I was already more familiar. I am a planner by nature but, for this exam, I would recommend some sort of timetable, no matter how approximate. And as everyone will tell you, Part 1 is a marathon not a sprint. Allow plenty of time. I planned to start revision in July (for a Part 1 exam in January) and, after a few false starts, finally got going in mid-September.

Everyone revises differently but here are my top three tips:

1. Delete social media – you will find there are plenty enough (more worthwhile – see point 3) things to do with any free moments. It's just not worth wasting that time checking Instagram.

2. Mix up the type of revision – I am primarily someone who learns by reading but I realised that I would need variety in order to maintain the revision momentum. I made notes (they are also useful to use for Part 2 later) and in between times practised questions. There are lots of question banks available but it's worth noting that none are specific to the FRCS (Urol). However, they can be useful in small measure for practising the art of answering an MCQ.

3. Take breaks – if you haven't quite left yourself enough time to cover everything then this might just be a short walk with a podcast, a quick gym session or a good TV show (but don't pick anything too addictive!). If you have planned well then make sure to make time for date night with your partner, a trip to the park with the kids or coffee with a friend and, if possible, have days with no or minimal revision.

Once you've sat in your (typically driving) test centre and passed your Part 1 there is often little time to turn around and prepare for Part 2 (unless you are planning a break or we hit another global pandemic that delays exams). Part 2 can be approached as more of a middle-distance race – eight weeks should be plenty of time (if you are attending the BAUS FRCS course then this is normally a reasonable time to start the big last push to the revision finish line). Take a decent break from the books and, if you can, go on holiday before starting revision again for Part 2.

The viva is about using the information you have from Part 1 and making sensible day-one urology consultant decisions. That's not to say that these are straightforward decisions – and the scenarios sometimes seem so improbable and uncommon that it's almost laughable. You wonder when you might actually need to know about emphysematous pyelonephritis or transuretero-ureterostomy, but trust me – I managed to encounter all 16 tables' worth of bizarre FRCS (Urol) scenarios during my first consultant on-call and have never been more grateful that I had sat the exam.

Revision for Part 2 is simple: practise, practise, practise (with a little bit of note revision and guideline reading – assuming you haven't immediately forgotten all of your Part 1 knowledge). Get a viva group together – aim for no more than three or four people at a time, but these can be drawn from a wider group. Aim to practise as often as you can – you can learn both from your own vivas as well as from vivaing others and observing others being viva'd, so make sure you make the most of every opportunity. Of course, work is like a perpetual FRCS exam: treat it as such, and make the most of the consultants and more senior trainees – say yes to any offer to be viva'd (no matter how embarrassing) and don't be afraid to ask for viva practice either. Courses are good but expensive in the main – if you can attend one this will help but don't feel like you must attend all of them.

Top three tips for the viva:

1. Listen to the question – if the question asks "how would you *manage* this patient" do not start talking about history/examination – the examiner wants to start straight with the first rung of the management ladder.

2. Try to learn history/exam/initial-investigation patter for key conditions of each table – this doesn't work all the time (for example, some scenarios start halfway through and technology is often just rapid-fire questions) but for most vivas it will give you a minute at the beginning of the station to recall the relevant information you need for the onward scenario, making the next nine minutes a bit easier.

3. Papers – there is no need to quote these ad nauseam. They need to be relevant and ideally only used to validate your decision making on more complex questions. Finally, only quote it if you really know it – examiners will rightly quiz you on it if you mention a paper. Save for a few key papers (mainly BPH and Oncology), knowledge of papers is not necessary to pass the FRCS.

People say you should enjoy the FRCS (Urol) viva, and if you do then congratulations – I didn't particularly. But preparing for this exam gives you the final pieces of the toolkit you will need for the rest of your consultant career – in a slightly perverse way, we should all be grateful for it. I wish you all good luck. Remember, "by failing to prepare, you prepare to fail" – so stop reading this and get reading the book!

Rachel Barratt

Keath Yeates Gold Medal Winner 2019
Consultant Urologist
UCLH

FOREWORD

I remember it like it was yesterday, that nauseating feeling of impending doom when I walked into the FRCS (Urol) examination hall to see what felt like an endless sea of examiners sat at tables, all eagerly awaiting to question me with varying degrees of intensity and ferocity. However, in hindsight, I've come to realise that in that brief moment of my career, I knew more about urology than I ever had done before or ever have done since. Arguably, the candidates sitting the FRCS (Urol) have a much wider depth of knowledge than many of the examiners, which is really quite an empowering feeling.

Now that you've opened this book, you have embarked on a journey that takes you to the end of your training career and the start of your consultant career. Inevitably, there are a mixture of feelings. For myself, there was nervous excitement at the thought of completing the final hurdle to commencing my consultant career. However, of course there was an overarching feeling of anxiety and fear: *"what if I fail?"*, *"who will employ me?"*, *"what are my next steps?"*. To reassure you, all of these thoughts and feelings are entirely normal for any candidate sitting any FRCS examination.

The FRCS (Urol) is an examination of two parts. The first is MCQ based, which requires the use of multiple resources. You can improve your pattern recognition by reviewing as many online or paper MCQs as you can find. Additionally, it's important to read well-known urology handbooks to ensure you have sufficient knowledge in common question themes, which include basic science, physiology, pharmacology, anatomy and urological nomenclature.

As I often say at the BAUS FRCS (Urol) viva course, my advice to all candidates for the second part of the FRCS (Urol) would be firstly to set up a viva group early with colleagues – ideally six-to-eight weeks before the exam. The magic number for your viva group is three, with one person to examine, one person to be the examinee and one person to give feedback. Secondly, get used to talking through scenarios, and practise, practise, practise. Unsurprisingly, the more you get used to talking through scenarios, the slicker and more polished you become. Never be too embarrassed to practise with people, no matter how good they say they are. Any experience is good experience. During the viva, always remember to take occasional pauses between your responses to allow time to gather your thoughts and invite the next question from the examiner. This way you can control the scenario and the pace of the examiner, which ultimately gives an impression of a confident and organised candidate. You will not know everything. If you don't know the answer on the day, don't be afraid to say "I'm afraid I can't recall" or "can I come back to that?". Again, this gives you control of the narrative and makes you appear relaxed and in control of the scenario (even though we know you'll be quaking in your boots under the table). Finally, never catastrophise; I can tell you now, you will more than likely have one "car crash" station where you feel you didn't represent yourself well. Compartmentalise this and move on. Each table is a new examiner who has no idea how your last station went, so you have a new opportunity to perform well.

Whilst the FRCS (Urol) is certainly a challenging and daunting experience, it is certainly a necessary rite of passage. You will find that you have developed more knowledge about the field of urology than you ever have done before. As a result, you will feel empowered and deserving of the coveted urology consultant appointment for which you have strived so hard for all these years.

Ultimately, this exam will be a nerve-racking experience. Try to remain calm, don't catastrophise and always ensure you are structured and safe in your responses. For what it's worth, try to enjoy the experience as much as you can, you will never know this much about urology ever again. One important thing to remember is that once you've completed the FRCS (Urol) the real challenge starts, which is actually convincing someone to give you a consultant job! Good luck and Godspeed.

Sotonye K. Tolofari BSc (Hons), MBChB, FRCS (Urol)

Keith Yeates Gold Medallist 2019
Consultant Urological Surgeon
Northern Care Alliance, Manchester

ACKNOWLEDGEMENTS

Compiling a more-than-600-page textbook is a rather time-consuming exercise, I have to say, and not straightforward to slot in between childcare and working as a full-time NHS consultant. Most of this textbook was written during night-time sessions between the hours of 10pm and 1am (or later). I therefore wish to apologise to everyone for having been more tired, strained and unsociable for the last six months.

I am indebted to Roger Amos and his team from Libri Publishing – without you this project would not have been possible, and you should be proud that you have had a key role in training future urologists around the world. Roger you are an absolute pleasure to work with and I hope we will collaborate on more projects together in the future.

I wish to thank Fiona McCaig for writing the renal transplantation chapter in Book 1. I appreciate you trying to sketch a dialysis machine the day after recovering from a late-night operation on a bleeding transplant kidney! Your contribution is invaluable and a great addition to the textbook.

I am very grateful to Rachel Barratt and Sot Tolofari for their forewords – it was very kind of you to share your advice and memories of the exam, and I am honoured that you both agreed to contribute to the textbook.

Thank you to my friends and colleagues for supporting me during a difficult time.

Thank you Shamah for all your love, care and attention for our son.

Thank you Mum for literally everything I can think of.

Thank you Dad. Unfortunately you never got to see the textbooks – but if indeed I do have any writing skills I am pretty sure they came from you.

And finally, thank you to my son, Zakariya – my love for you has changed the whole way I live and view life since you came along. You are a beautiful shining star and I am proud of you every day.

INTRODUCTION

Dear colleague, thank you so much for choosing the second edition of *Essential Revision Notes for the FRCS (Urol)*. I sincerely hope it serves you as a valuable, helpful and trustworthy companion throughout the long odyssey that is the FRCS (Urol), and that ultimately the book supports you in passing the exam.

I wish to briefly share with you the story behind the first and second editions of my book, for some light-heartedness prior to hundreds of pages of facts and figures.

As I began to prepare and write my personal revision notes for the FRCS (Urol), within no more than a week the idea came to me that as (all being well) I would likely be sat at the same desk revising for the best part of seven months, I might as well construct and format my notes as I studied along the way such that by the end of the process I would have a manuscript ready for publication. By the end I even had it neatly printed, bound and laminated ready to present to a publishing company.

As it happened, the euphoria of passing the exam, then moving house and general life busyness resulted in the manuscript being put in a box (but fortunately not being lost in the house move) and in my heart I gave up on the idea of publishing it. Ultimately I was simply grateful that I had passed the exam.

When the COVID-19 pandemic struck, however, between self-isolation, lockdowns, support bubbles and erratic work rotas I found myself unexpectedly having extended periods of time at home. I found the box with the manuscript. I recall literally blowing dust off the top of it. I went about organising interviews with various publishers until Roger Amos and John Sivak from Libri Publishing saved the day – and the rest is history.

The tentative first-edition project proved to be more successful than we would have ever imagined and above all the feedback I got from colleagues was that they found my book handy for their revision and were grateful. (However, from a financial point of view I do not recommend becoming a writer of medical textbooks – stick to being a doctor!)

The fact that I knew I had helped people made the production of a second edition imperative.

The atmosphere in my mind when writing the second edition was different – this is because whilst producing the first edition we were expecting our son, Zakariya. I thus felt I had a race against time to complete as I presumed that, once he was born, I would barely have time to eat – and I was right. This time round therefore, as he was now more grown up, I thought I would have more free time and spare energy – but I was wrong. Parenting does not get any easier!

In order to ensure I would be providing as accurate, tidy, relevant and up-to-date information as possible to my colleagues, I committed to painstakingly reviewing every single word, line and punctuation mark you will find in the book. This took a *lot* longer than I had anticipated.

Not that I think I have quite reached a stage where I can compare myself to Leonardo da Vinci just yet; but the best comparison I can make of the contrast between the production of the two editions is with his painting of the Last Supper – about three years to paint it (first edition) and more than 21 years for its restoration (second edition).

So here I present to you, only eight months contractually late (sorry Roger), the completed second edition of *Essential Revision Notes for the FRCS (Urol)*.

There are many new features in this edition that I really hope you will find helpful:

- All information robustly fact-checked, with relevant NICE and EAU guidance up-to-date as of 2024
- More than 170 new sample MCQs
- Bonus chapter "Viva Tips & Tricks", where I share my advice having been faculty member on multiple different FRCS (Urol) revision courses over the years
- Bonus chapter "Renal Transplantation", which I wish to thank Fiona McCaig for writing, as I felt it more appropriate for an expert in the field to be entrusted to guide you with what you need to know on this topic
- Important scientific papers for you to be aware of and read up about are now highlighted with the symbol $\boxed{\text{KEY PAPER}}$, with 17 additional papers featuring in the book as well as those present in the first edition
- I share practical advice for the FRCS (Urol) viva section, which can be identified with the symbol $\boxed{\text{VIVA}}$, with 48 of these now featuring
- Errata corrige (thank you to those who contacted me highlighting any mistakes in the first edition)
- More consistent, succinct and fluent reading style.

As ever I recommend that you use this book as the roadmap/skeleton for your revision. You cannot pass the FRCS (Urol) using a single resource, however: you must complement this with other textbooks, courses and online material.

I am very grateful to Rachel Barratt and Sot Tolofari for their invaluable contributions to the book with their advice on how to master the FRCS (Urol) – as Gold Medal winners you really ought to follow their recommendations on that rather than mine.

I would, however, wish to briefly share with you my thoughts, memories and advice on the FRCS (Urol) journey.

It is a long expedition. Clear the mental deck if you can – by which I mean avoid taking the exam at the same time as major life events like getting married or moving house. Start revising early (I began three months before Section 1). Talk to as many colleagues as you can who have recently passed the exam to find common themes in how they did it and what resources they used. Do not cram – if someone tells you they successfully did that, it probably isn't true. Vary your revision to keep you engaged – you can read notes, watch videos, practise MCQs, use flash cards. For the viva section, it is all about practice – form a small revision group and commit to practising every evening if possible, from the moment after attending the BAUS FRCS (Urol) revision course.

Above all, try to enjoy it. This should be your last hurdle after having completed innumerable exams to reach the end of your surgical training, and arguably all the information you will learn and absorb during the FRCS (Urol) journey will be relevant to your future practice as a urologist. You will hopefully be interested to discover the evidence behind a lot of the practice you currently do (many trainees, like me before, mostly know what they should do but not *why* they do it) and you will hopefully enjoy the feeling of really finally *knowing your stuff*.

Having expertise to be able to help a sick patient in their time of need is truly a gift. This consideration galvanised me to master the FRCS (Urol) exam and continues to motivate me to keep improving my practice as a doctor every day, to learn more, do more, serve more and teach more. I hope this will inspire you.

I do wish you all the very best.

Jack Donati-Bourne

GLOSSARY OF ABBREVIATIONS

AAST – American Association for the Surgery of Trauma
ABU – anastomotic bulbar urethroplasty
ACEi – angiotensin converting enzyme inhibitor
ACR – albumin creatinine ratio
ACT – α1 anti-chymotrypsin
ACTH – adreno-corticotropic hormone
ADC – apparent diffusion coefficient
ADH – anti-diuretic hormone
ADT – androgen deprivation therapy
AFP – alpha feto-protein
AKI – acute kidney injury
ALP – alkaline phosphatase
ALPP – abdominal leak-point pressure
AMG – α2 macro globulin
AML – angiomyolipoma
AP – antero-posterior
APC – adenomatous polyposis coli
APD – antero-posterior diameter
APLS – Advanced Paediatric Life Support
ARR – absolute risk reduction
AS – active surveillance
ASAP – atypical small acinar proliferation
ATLS – Advanced Trauma Life Support
ATN – acute tubular necrosis
ATP – adenosine triphosphate
AUA – American Urology Association
AUR – acute urinary retention
AUS – artificial urethral sphincter
AVF – arterio-venous fistula
BAPU – British Association of Paediatric Urologists
BAUS – British Association of Urological Surgeons
BCG – Bacillus Calmette–Guerin
BCI – bladder contractility index
BHD – Birt–Hogg–Dubé
BMD – bone mineral density
BNF – British National Formulary
BNI – bladder neck incision
BOO – bladder outlet obstruction

BOOI – bladder outlet obstruction index
BPE – benign prostatic enlargement
BPH – benign prostatic hyperplasia
BPS – bladder pain syndrome
BTB – blood–testis barrier
BTx – brachytherapy
BXO – balanitis xerotica obliterans
CAH – congenital adrenal hyperplasia
CAIS – complete androgen insensitivity syndrome
CAP – continuous antibiotic prophylaxis
CAPD – continuous ambulatory peritoneal dialysis
CBAVD – congenital bilateral absence of vas deferens
CBP – chronic bacterial prostatitis
CCG – clinical commissioning group
CCI – Charlson Comorbidity Index
CCrISP – Care of the Critically Ill Surgical Patient
CF – cystic fibrosis
CFU – colony forming units
cGMP – cyclic guanosine monophosphate
CI – confidence interval
CIS – carcinoma in situ
CKD – chronic kidney disease
CMV – cytomegalovirus
CN – cytoreductive nephrectomy
CNS – central nervous system
COPD – chronic obstructive pulmonary disease
CPEX – cardio-pulmonary exercise testing
CPG – Cambridge prognostic group
CPPS – chronic pelvic pain syndrome
CRP – C-reactive protein
CRPC – castrate resistant prostate cancer
CSF – cerebrospinal fluid
CSS – cancer specific survival
CT – computed tomography
CT TAP – computed tomography of thorax abdomen and pelvis
CTU – computed tomography urogram
CVA – cerebrovascular accident
CVVH – continuous veno-venous haemofiltration
CXR – chest x-ray
DCE – dynamic contrast enhanced
DEXA – dual energy absorptiometry scan

DFS – disease-free survival
DHT – dihydrotestosterone
DLPP – detrusor leak-point pressure
DMSA – dimercaptosuccinic acid
DNA – deoxyribonucleic acid
DO – detrusor overactivity
DRE – digital rectal examination
DetSD – detrusor sphincter dyssynergia
DSD – differences in sex development
DSNB – dynamic sentinel node biopsy
DTPA – diethylene-triamine-pentaacetate
DVC – dorsal venous complex
DVT – deep-vein thrombosis
DWI-MRI – diffusion-weighted magnetic resonance imaging
EAU – European Association Urology
EBL – estimated blood loss
EBRT – external beam radiotherapy
ECG – electro-cardiogram
ECOG – Eastern Cooperative Oncology Group
ED – erectile dysfunction
EDTA – ethylenediaminetetraacetic acid
EMA – European Medicines Agency
EMRT – emergency medical response team
EORTC – European Organisation for Research and Treatment of Cancer
EPE – extra-prostatic extension
EPLND – extended pelvic lymph-node dissection
EPN – emphysematous pyelonephritis
EPO – erythropoietin
EPR – extra-peritoneal
ERSPC – European Randomised Study of Screening for Prostate Cancer
ESRF – end-stage renal failure
ESWL – extra-corporeal shockwave lithotripsy
ETS – E26 transformation specific
EUA – examination under anaesthesia
FBC – full blood count
FDA – Food and Drug Administration
FDG – fluorodeoxyglucose
FFP – fresh frozen plasma
FNA – fine-needle aspiration
FSGS – focal segmental glomerulosclerosis
FSH – follicle stimulating hormone

FUD – female urethral diverticulum
FURS – flexible ureteroscopy
FVC – frequency–volume chart
f/t PSA – free to total prostate-specific antigen
GA – general anaesthesia
GAG – glycosaminoglycans
GCNIS – germ cell neoplasia in situ
GCS – Glasgow coma scale
GCT – germ cell tumour
GFR – glomerular filtration rate
GnRH – gonadotropin-releasing hormone
GS – Gram stain
GTN – glyceryl trinitrate
GUCG – Genito-Urinary Cancer Group
HDL – high-density lipoprotein
HDP – hydroxydiphosphonate
HEPA – high-efficiency particulate air
HFEA – Human Fertilisation and Embryology Authority
HG – high grade
HGPIN – high-grade prostatic intra-epithelial neoplasia
HIF – hypoxia-inducible factor
HIFU – high-intensity focused ultrasound
HIV – human immunodeficiency virus
HK – human kallikrein
HLA – human leucocyte antigen
HLRCC – hereditary leiomyomatosis and renal cell carcinoma
HoLEP – holmium laser enucleation of the prostate
HPCRU – high-pressure chronic retention of urine
HPF – high-powered field
HPG – hypothalamo–pituitary–gonadal
HPRC – hereditary papillary renal carcinoma
HPV – human papilloma virus
HU – Hounsfield unit
IBD – inflammatory bowel disease
ICCS – International Children's Continence Society
ICD – implanted cardiac defibrillator
ICIQ-UI – International Consultation on Incontinence Questionnaire
ICS – International Continence Society
ICSI – intra-cytoplasmic sperm injection
IDO – idiopathic detrusor overactivity
IGCCCG – International Germ Cell Cancer Collaborative Group

IGF – insulin growth factor
IHD – ischaemic heart disease
IHT – intermittent hormone therapy
IIEF – International Index of Erectile Function
IM – intra-muscular
IMRT – intensity-modulated radiation therapy
INR – international normalised ratio
IPR – intra-peritoneal
IPSS – International Prostate Symptom Score
IR – interventional radiology
ISC – intermittent self-catheterisation
ISD – intermittent self-dilatation
ISUP – International Society of Urological Pathology
ITGCN – intra-tubular germ cell neoplasia
ITU – intensive therapy unit
IUI – intra-uterine insemination
IV – intra-venous
IVC – inferior vena cava
IVF – in-vitro fertilisation
IVU – intra-venous urogram
kD – kilo Dalton
KSS – kidney-sparing surgery
KUB – kidneys ureter bladder
LASER – light amplification by stimulated emission of radiation
LDL – low-density lipoprotein
LFT – liver function tests
LG – low grade
LH – luteinising hormone
LHRH – luteinising hormone releasing hormone
LN – lymph node
LND – lymph-node dissection
LOH – late onset hypogonadism
LOS – length of stay
LTC – long-term catheter
LUT – lower urinary tract
LUTD – lower urinary tract dysfunction
LUTS – lower urinary tract symptoms
LVI – lympho-vascular invasion
MAB – maximum androgen blockade
MAG3 – mercapto acetyltriglycine
MAP – mean arterial pressure

MCDK – multi-cystic dysplastic kidney
mCRPC – metastatic castrate resistant prostate cancer
MCUG – micturating cysto-urethrogram
MDP – methylene diphosphonate
MDRD – Modification of Diet in Renal Disease
MDT – multi-disciplinary team
MET – medical expulsive therapy
mg – milligram
MHRA – Medicines and Healthcare products Regulatory Agency
MHz – megahertz
MI – myocardial infarction
MIBC – muscle-invasive bladder cancer
MIBG – metaiodobenzylguanidine
MIS – Mullerian inhibiting substance
mL – millilitre
MMC – mitomycin-C
MNE – monosymptomatic nocturnal enuresis
mPCa – metastatic prostate cancer
mpMRI – multi-parametric magnetic resonance imaging
mRCC – metastatic renal cell carcinoma
MRI – magnetic resonance imaging
MRU – magnetic resonance urogram
MS – multiple sclerosis
MSU – midstream urine
MUI – mixed urinary incontinence
MV – megavoltage
NA – noradrenaline
NAAT – nucleic acid amplification test
NAC – neo-adjuvant chemotherapy
NBI – narrow-band imaging
NCCT – non-contrast computed tomography
Nd – neodymium
NDO – neurogenic detrusor overactivity
NEWS2 – National Early Warning Score 2
ng – nanogram
NGT – nasogastric tube
NHS – National Health Service
NICE – National Institute of Clinical Excellence
NICU – neonatal intensive care unit
NIDDK – National Institute of Diabetes, Digestive and Kidney Diseases
NMIBC – non-muscle-invasive bladder cancer

NNS – number needed to screen
NNT – number needed to treat
NO – nitric oxide
NPV – negative predictive value
NS – nerve sparing
NSAID – non-steroidal anti-inflammatory drug
NSGCT – non-seminomatous germ cell tumour
NVB – neurovascular bundle
NVH – non-visible haematuria
OAB – overactive bladder
OD – once daily
OS – overall survival
PAE – prostate artery embolisation
PCa – prostate cancer
PCN – percutaneous nephrostomy
PCNL – percutaneous nephrolithotomy
PDD – photo dynamic diagnosis
PDE5i – phosphodiesterase-5 inhibitor
PDGF – platelet-derived growth factor
PE – pulmonary embolism
PeIN – penile intraepithelial neoplasia
PET – positron emission tomography
PID – pelvic inflammatory disease
PI-RADS – Prostate Imaging Reporting and Data System
PFE – pelvic-floor exercises
PFMT – pelvic-floor muscle training
PFS – progression free survival
PFUDD – pelvic fracture urethral distraction defects
PGE$_1$ – prostaglandin E$_1$
PGF$_2$ – prostaglandin F$_2$
PN – partial nephrectomy
PO – per oral
POP – pelvic organ prolapse
PPI – proton pump inhibitor
PPS – prostate pain syndrome
PPV – patent processus vaginalis
PR – per rectum
PRN – pro re nata
PSA – prostate-specific antigen
PSAD – prostate-specific antigen density
PSADT – prostate-specific antigen doubling time

PSATZD – prostate-specific antigen transitional zone density
PSAV – prostate-specific antigen velocity
PSMA – prostate-specific membrane antigen
PTFE – polytetrafluoroethane
PTH – parathyroid hormone
PTLD – post-transplant lympho-proliferative disease
PTNS – posterior tibial nerve stimulation
PUJ – pelviureteric junction
PUJO – pelviureteric junction obstruction
PUNLMP – papillary urothelial neoplasm of low malignant potential
PUV – posterior urethral valves
PVD – peripheral vascular disease
PVR – post-void residual
QDS – quarter die sumendum (four times daily)
QOL – quality of life
qSOFA – quick sepsis-related organ failure assessment
RBC – red blood cell
RCC – renal cell carcinoma
RCT – randomised controlled trial
RFA – radio-frequency ablation
RN – radical nephrectomy
RNA – ribonucleic acid
RNU – radical nephroureterectomy
RP – radical prostatectomy
RR – relative risk
RRT – renal replacement therapy
RTA – renal tubular acidosis
RTB – renal tumour biopsy
RTx – radiotherapy
RU – retrograde urethrography
rUTI – recurrent urinary tract infection
SCC – spinal cord compression
SCCa – squamous cell carcinoma
SCI – spinal cord injury
SD – standard deviation
SFR – stone-free rate
SHBG – sex hormone binding globulin
SIADH – syndrome of inappropriate secretion of anti-diuretic hormone
SIRS – systemic inflammatory response syndrome
SNM – sacral neuromodulation
SOFA – sequential organ failure assessment

SPC – suprapubic catheter
SPECT – single-photon emission computed tomography
sPSA – super-sensitive prostate-specific antigen
SRM – small renal mass
SSRI – selective serotonin reuptake inhibitor
STI – sexually transmitted infection
SUI – stress urinary incontinence
Sv – sievert
TB – tuberculosis
Tc – technetium
TC – testicular cancer
TCC – transitional cell carcinoma
TDS – ter die sumendum (three times daily)
TENS – trans-cutaneous electrical nerve stimulation
TESE – testicular sperm extraction
TIN – testicular intra-epithelial neoplasia
TKI – tyrosine kinase inhibitor
TLR – toll-like receptor
TMPRSS2 – trans-membrane protease serine 2
TOT – trans-obturator tape
TPN – total parenteral nutrition
TRT – testosterone replacement therapy
TRUS – trans-rectal ultrasound
TSG – tumour suppressor gene
TUIP – trans-urethral incision of prostate
TURBT – trans-urethral resection of bladder tumour
TURED – trans-urethral resection of ejaculatory ducts
TURP – trans-urethral resection of prostate
TVT – tension-free vaginal tape
UDS – urodynamics
UDT – undescended testis
UE – urea and electrolytes
ULD – ultra low-dose
URS – ureteroscopy
US – ultrasound
USA – United States of America
USANZ – Urological Society of Australia and New Zealand
UTI – urinary tract infection
UTUC – upper-tract urothelial cancer
UUI – urge urinary incontinence
VEGF – vascular endothelial growth factor

VH – visible haematuria
VHL – Von Hippel–Lindau syndrome
VIP – vaso-active intestinal peptide
VI-RADS – Vesical Imaging-Reporting and Data System
VLPP – Valsalva leak-point pressure
VTE – venous thrombo-embolism
VUDS – video urodynamics
VUJ – vesico-ureteric junction
VUR – vesico-ureteric reflux
VVF – vesicovaginal fistula
WCC – white cell count
WHO – World Health Organization
WLE – wide local excision
WW – watchful waiting
XGP – xanthogranulomatous pyelonephritis
XR – x-ray
YAG – yttrium aluminium garnet
ZA – zoledronic acid
5-ALA – 5-aminolaevulinic acid
5AR – 5-alpha reductase
5ARIs – 5-alpha reductase inhibitors
5-FU – 5-fluorouracil

STATION 5
CALCULI & URINARY TRACT INFECTIONS

STONES: BROAD PRINCIPLES

EPIDEMIOLOGY

Lifetime risk in developed countries is ~10% and the incidence is rising.

Men at higher risk; however, risk is equalising with women due to obesity/dietary trends in society.

Recurrence rates are quoted ≤ 50%.

Age 30–60 years is the peak incidence for stone formation.

RISK FACTORS

Intrinsic Factors:

- *Gender* – men at higher risk (testosterone increases oxalate production in liver) (women have higher urinary citrate concentration which inhibits calcium oxalate stone formation)
- *Genetic* – most common in Caucasian people
- *Diseases* – e.g. hyperparathyroidism, polycystic kidney disease, Crohn's and malabsorption pathologies, obesity/bariatric surgery, gout
- *Neurological* – such as MS, SCI (bone demineralisation), neurogenic bladder
- Anatomy – increased risk with PUJO and horseshoe kidney
- *UTIs* – due to urease-producing bacteria (Proteus, Klebsiella, Enterobacter)
- *Drugs* – corticosteroids (increased gut calcium absorption), chemotherapy [1]

Extrinsic Factors:

- *Geographical* – for example Middle-East stone belt
- *Seasonal* – more common in hotter months (peak is one month after summer)
- *Dietary* – including high salt and protein intake, low water intake, <u>low</u> calcium intake

CLASSIFICATION

There are many different ways of classifying stones.

These include according to composition, x-ray appearance, size, location, risk of recurrence, aetiology of formation, infection vs. non-infectious causes.

Stone Composition

Calcium oxalate stones are the most common type of kidney stone.

A summary of the different types of urinary tract stones is shown in Table 1.

80% of uric acid stones are pure, 20% are mixed containing calcium oxalate.

The proteinaceous portion of stones is composed of matrix (depending on stone type, kidney stones contain 2.5–65% of non-crystalline matrix).

Stone composition is covered further in this chapter in "Stone Compositions" below.

Table 1 – Summary of different composition of urinary tract stones

Stone Composition	% of All Stones	Aetiological Classification
Calcium oxalate	80	
Uric acid	10	Non-infection stone
Calcium phosphate + oxalate	10	
Struvite (infection/triple phosphate stones)	10	Infection stone
Cystine	1	Genetic causes
Xanthine	Rare	
Indinavir, triamterene	Rare	Drug stones

Radiodensity on X-ray

Three broad categories of stones are described based on their x-ray appearance (Table 2).

The degree of a stone's radio-opacity on plain-film XR can provide some indication of its composition and thus guide treatment options.

Measuring the HU on CT KUB, however, provides more reliable information regarding density.

Table 2 – Categories of urinary tract stones based on their x-ray appearance

X-ray Appearance	Composition
Radio-opaque	Calcium oxalate, calcium phosphate
Poor radio-opacity	cystine, magnesium ammonium phosphate (struvite)
Radio-lucent	Uric acid, drug stones (not visible on CT KUB), xanthine

Stone Size and Location

Guidelines use linear measurement of cumulative diameters to stratify stones into following groups:

- < 5mm; 5–10mm; 10–20mm; > 20mm (for use in treatment algorithm).

Stones can also be classified according to their anatomical position:

- *Renal*: upper/middle/lower calyx or renal pelvis
- *Ureter*: upper/mid/lower ureter
- *Bladder*.

Prostatic calculi are usually asymptomatic, they do not affect PSA readings and are made of calcium phosphate/carbonate. [2]

Urethral stones are uncommon, and in women are often associated with urethral diverticulum.

STONE FORMATION

Solubility product (Ksp) refers to the point of saturation where dissolved and crystalline components in solution are in equilibrium.

The driving force behind stone formation is the supersaturation of urine.

Supersaturation occurs when product of concentrations of salts exceeds Ksp.

Supersaturation is expressed as ratio of urinary mineral (e.g. calcium oxalate) to solubility, where (supersaturation < 1) = crystals remain soluble, (supersaturation > 1) = crystals nucleate/grow.

Above Ksp however, crystals still do not form spontaneously due to inhibitors of formation (although crystallisation can occur on top of pre-existing crystals).

This condition is called the *metastable state*.

However, above a certain concentration of salts the inhibitors no longer function and crystals start forming spontaneously.

The concentration above which this process begins to happen is formation product (Kf). [3]

Urine with concentration between Ksp and Kf is defined as *metastable*.

Summary of principles using calcium oxalate as an example:

- calcium + oxalate concentration < Ksp   -> no stone formation
- calcium + oxalate concentration = metastable   -> no stone formation
- calcium + oxalate concentration > Kf   -> stone formation

The process by which nuclei form in pure solutions is called *homogenous nucleation*.

The state of saturation of the urine (*saturation index*) with respect to particular stone-forming salts indicates the stone-forming propensity of the urine.

Epitaxy

The deposition of one type of crystal upon the surface of another crystal of different composition but similar lattice structure is known as epitaxy.

Uric acid crystals may promote superimposed calcium oxalate stone formation (however, rarely cystine).

Randall's Plaques

Although urine is not usually supersaturated with calcium, this may occur in the loop of Henle, leading to precipitation of calcium phosphate in interstitial sites in the inner medulla.

These deposits may develop to the extent that they become visible – these are *Randall's plaques*.

These plaques have been proposed to act as nidus for development of calcium oxalate stones. [4]

Inhibitors of Crystallisation

Citrate is the only inhibitor of stone formation that is open to manipulation.

Citrate forms soluble complex with calcium, preventing it combining with oxalate/phosphate to agglomerate into crystals.

Citrate therefore lowers the urinary saturation of calcium oxalate.

Primary determinant of urinary citrate excretion is acid–base status (metabolic acidosis reduces citrate excretion as it is metabolised to bicarbonate; alkalosis increases excretion).

Other inhibitors include Tamm–Horsfall proteins, magnesium, GAG, prothrombin fragment 1.

STONE COMPOSITIONS

CALCIUM OXALATE STONES

Most patients with calcium oxalate stones have ≥ 1 metabolic abnormality (e.g. hypercalciuria, hyperoxaluria) but in most cases the cause of the abnormality itself is unknown.

The associated metabolic abnormalities are further detailed under the relevant sub-headings below.

Low urine volume is the most important predisposing factor to formation of calcium oxalate stones.

Calcium oxalate stones can exist at monohydrate (*whewellite*) and dihydrate (*weddellite*).

Calcium oxalate monohydrate stones are much harder to break – crystals are dumbbell-shaped.

Calcium oxalate dihydrate crystals are pyramidal-shaped.

| VIVA | Questions around the different shapes of kidney stones under microscopy are FRCS (Urol) favourites, both in the written and viva sections. I recommend you ensure you can name the particular stone type if you are shown a microscopy slide of a kidney stone.

Hypercalciuria

Hypercalciuria is defined as excretion of > 300mg (men) or > 250mg (women) of urine calcium per day.

This increases supersaturation of urine, and can be due to calcium:

- Absorption, (i.e. increased in intestine) seen in *absorptive hypercalciuria*
- Excretion, due to leakage from kidney
- Resorption, due to increased bone demineralisation.

The vitamin-D metabolite that stimulates intestinal calcium absorption is 1,25-dihydroxyvitamin D3.

Renal leak hypercalciuria:

- Is due to renal wasting of calcium due to impairment of renal tubular calcium reabsorption
- Eventually leads to secondary hyperparathyroidism (low bone density)
- Is treated with thiazide diuretics (augments calcium reabsorption in proximal tubule).

Hypercalcaemia

Raised serum levels of calcium increase the risk of stone formation in patients.

There are many potential causes of hypercalcaemia; most common reasons include underlying primary hyperparathyroidism or cancers.

Medications such as thiazide diuretics and vitamin-D supplements may also raise serum calcium.

Management of hypercalcaemia in elective setting involves finding and treating the underlying cause.

Hyperoxaluria

Increased oxalate in the urine can arise from:

- Leakage, via altered membrane transport leading to increased renal loss
- Over-production, primary cause in liver
- Excessive absorption, increased oxalate absorption in bowel.

The primary site of intestinal absorption of oxalate is in the large bowel.

Enteric hyperoxaluria is managed by calcium supplements (these bind excess oxalate within intestine which is soluble), potassium citrate (inhibitory stone formation) and increase fluid intake.

Hyperoxaluria is the most common urinary finding in patients who have had gastric bypass surgery.

Intestinal oxalate absorption is modulated by diet – low dietary calcium increases oxalate absorption due to reduced formation of soluble calcium-oxalate complex lost in stool.

O.formigenes is an oxalate-degrading bacterium found in intestinal lumen that uses oxalate as energy source, thereby reducing its absorption and thus urinary oxalate concentration.

Aetiology of stone formation in cystic fibrosis patients is due to reduced/absent O.formigenes.

In IBD the intestinal fat malabsorption increases calcium soap formation, limiting the amount free to complex with oxalate which in turn is free for absorption. [5]

Other Metabolic Abnormalities

Hypocitraturia, as citrate is stone-inhibitor (causes include renal tubular acidosis, hypokalaemia), managed by increased fluid and citrus fruit intake, potassium citrate supplementation.

Hyperuricosuria, high urinary uric acid levels, which can be managed with allopurinol.

URIC ACID STONES

Approximately 50% of patients with uric acid stones have gout (20% of gout patients get stones).

The rest are idiopathic or due to myeloproliferative disorders and their cytotoxic treatment (cell necrosis releases large amounts of nucleic acids converted to uric acid).

There are no known inhibitors of uric acid crystallisation.

Urine is supersaturated with insoluble uric acid.

Uric acid exists in two forms in urine: uric acid (insoluble) and sodium urate (20x more soluble).

As the pH rises, the proportion of uric acid as sodium urate increases, thus increasing the overall solubility (i.e. acidic low urinary pH predisposes to uric acid stone formation).

Uric acid stones are the only ones reliably dissolved by medical agents (e.g. potassium citrate).

Potassium citrate (rather than sodium bicarbonate) is preferred as alkalinising agent as the sodium may inhibit calcium reabsorption, leading to hypercalciuria and thus calcium oxalate stone formation.

Diet is important in prevention – high protein/purine increases uric acid excretion and lowers pH.

Under light microscopy, uric acid crystals appear rectangular.

Figure 1 – Uric acid formation and summary of stone prevention strategies

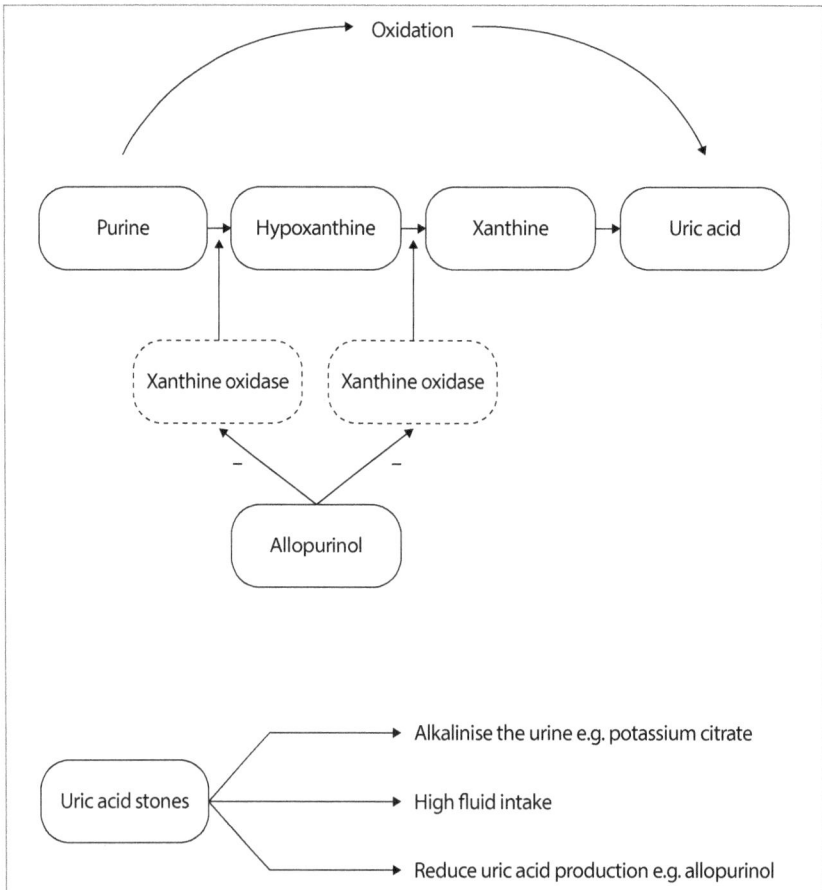

STRUVITE STONES

Struvite stones are composed of magnesium, ammonium and phosphate (i.e. triple phosphate).

Urease-producing bacteria breakdown urea into ammonia, which alkalinises the urine increasing crystal precipitation of magnesium, ammonium and phosphate.

Struvite crystals look like coffin lids under microscopy.

Acetohydroxamic acid is a competitive inhibitor of urease enzyme and can be given to prevent stone recurrence in patients with chronic urea-splitting infections.

Its use is limited by side-effects including DVT risk, hair loss and haemolytic anaemia.

IMAGING

After appropriate history and clinical examination, if ureteric colic is suspected then imaging will be required to further evaluate.

NICE 2019 guidance for diagnostic imaging in urolithiasis is as follows: [6]

- Offer urgent (within 24 hours of presentation) low-dose non-contrast CT to adults with suspected renal colic; if a woman is pregnant, offer US instead of CT
- Offer urgent (within 24 hours of presentation) US as first-line imaging for children/young people with suspected renal colic
- If uncertainty remains about the diagnosis of renal colic after US for children/young people, consider low-dose non-contrast CT.

Remember in children adopt the ALARA radiation approach (As Low As Reasonably Achievable).

US URINARY TRACT

US is a safe and inexpensive imaging tool – modality of choice in pregnancy and children.

US can detect stones in kidney, VUJ (with filled bladder) and upper-tract dilatation.

Sensitivity of ~45% for both ureteric and kidney stones, and a specificity for kidney (88%) and ureteric stones (94%) and may even avoid need for CT in many patients.

NON-CONTRAST CT KUB

CT KUB is standard for diagnosing acute flank pain (replacing old IVU) and provides information regarding stone location, size, skin-to-stone distance, HU.

Sensitivity is 94–100% and specificity is 92–100%.

No contrast is required and therefore no cut-off GFR applicable.

Indinavir stones and pure matrix stones (protein and cellular debris) are radio-lucent stones on CT.

Recommend to scan prone – VUJ stones that have passed into bladder will fall away from VUJ.

Standard CT KUB radiation dose is 4.7mSv (IVU is 3mSv).

Natural incidence of fatal cancer is 1 in 5; a 10mSv dose increases this by 1 in 2,000, therefore a CT KUB by 1 in 4,000.

Alternative option is ULD CT KUB with dose 2–3mSv; however, this is at the expense of lower sensitivity.

CT Signs of Obstruction

The signs of obstruction on CT KUB include: [7]

- Hydronephrosis and/or increased renal size (nephromegaly)
- Unilateral peri-nephrite/ureteric stranding
- Ureteric wall oedema/ring around the stone (*rim sign*).

Hounsfield Unit

HU is a quantitative scale for measuring radiodensity.

Zero HU is the radiodensity of distilled water at standard pressure and temperature. The HU of other common substances in the body are shown in Table 3.

Table 3 – Hounsfield unit values for different substances in the body [7]

Substance	HU on CT
Air	-1,000
Lung	-500
Fat	-100 to -50
Water	0
Kidney	30
Muscle	10 to 40
Bone	700 (cancellous) to 3,000 (cortical)

HU have ability to predict stone composition and thus help determine effective management plan for treating individual patient.

Uric acid stones have low density (e.g. 200–450HU) and can be treated with urine alkalinisation.

Calcium-bases stones have higher density ($\geq$ 1,000HU) making them more resistant to ESWL and more likely to require surgical intervention.

CT attenuation values prior to ESWL helps predict treatment success:

- Threshold of $\leq$ 815HU has significantly better stone clearance rates. [8]

The attenuation values of common stone composition types are shown in Table 4.

Table 4 – HU for different compositions of stones [7]

Stone Composition	Hounsfield Units
Uric acid	200–450
Struvite	600–900
Cystine	600–1,100
Calcium phosphate	1,200–1,600

XR KUB

XR KUB should not be routinely performed in addition to CT KUB.

Sensitivity is 45% and specificity is 80%.

XR KUB can be useful in determining radio-opaque vs. radio-lucent, and valid tool for follow-up purposes for radio-opaque stones.

MR UROGRAM

MRU cannot be used to identify ureteric stones; however, it can provide information regarding the level of obstruction, hydronephrosis and renal parenchymal morphology. [9]

Stones may be visualised as filling defects.

EAU 2024 recommends MRU as second-line investigation for ureteric colic in pregnant women after US.

METABOLIC EVALUATION

There is no established consensus as to how stone formers should be evaluated metabolically.

Stone analysis (performed by infra-red spectroscopy or XR diffraction) should ideally be performed in all first-time stone formers.

One method is to determine patient's risk of recurrence after stone passage, such that high-risk patients undergo thorough work-up, whilst low-risk patients have abbreviated work-up.

Low-risk metabolic work-up includes:

- *Blood tests*, UEs, serum urate/calcium/phosphate
- *Urinalysis*, including pH, culture and sensitivity for bacteria, microscopy for crystals
- *Stone analysis*.

Factors that may deem a patient to be at higher risk of recurrent stone formation:

- Children (EAU 2024 recommends completing a metabolic evaluation in all children)
- Significant family history
- Recurrent stone formers and/or short interval since last episode

- History of gout, recurrent UTIs, bowel malabsorption, osteoporosis
- Staghorn calculi or multiple bilateral calculi.

High-risk metabolic work-up includes (in addition to low-risk work-up): [7]

- 24-hour urine collection
- Dietary diary.

24-hour Urine Collection

Discard first voided urine, then start test: collect all urine including following morning's first voided one.

Store at cool temperature to prevent crystallisation; return to the lab for analysis as soon as possible.

Two 24-hour urine collections are recommended as standard:

1. Bottle with hydrochloric acid (tests 24-hour calcium, oxalate, phosphate, citrate)
2. Standard bottle (tests 24-hour uric acid, electrolytes, pH, urine volume).

PAIN RELIEF

NSAIDs are first-line analgesic drug for acute ureteric colic advised by NICE and EAU 2024. [10]

NICE advises IV paracetamol should be used second line, or first line if NSAID contraindicated. [6]

NSAIDs have better analgesic efficacy than opioids, and are less likely to require rescue analgesia in the short term, and opioids are associated with higher incidence of nausea and vomiting. [11]

NSAIDs induce afferent arteriole vasoconstriction mediated by prostaglandins, which reduce diuresis, oedema and smooth muscle stimulation.

The addition of anti-spasmodics to NSAIDs does not improve pain control.

URETERIC STENT VS. NEPHROSTOMY

An infected obstructed kidney is a urological emergency.

The patient should be resuscitated in a systematic Airway-to-Exposure manner, completing the Sepsis-6 bundle, keeping the patient fasted and involving outreach/critical care.

CT KUB should be obtained urgently to confirm the diagnosis of obstructing stone.

There are two main options for urgent decompression of an infected obstructed kidney:

- Placement of retrograde ureteric stent
- Insertion of PCN.

Studies suggest the two methods are equally effective in relieving the obstruction/infection.

For example a study randomising 42 patients presenting with obstructing ureteric calculi and infection to either PCN or retrograde ureteric stenting found: [12]

- Time to treatment was comparable between the two groups
- Time to normal temperature was 2.3 days (nephrostomy) vs. 2.6 days (stent).

The decision may be based on logistical factors, surgeon preference and stone characteristics.

EAU 2024 recommends PCN or stenting are both suitable options in the emergency context.

Table 5 – Percutaneous nephrostomy vs. retrograde ureteric stenting [7]

Factor	Stent vs. PCN (Pros and Cons)
Nephrostomy bag	None required for stent
Failure rate	Lower in PCN (impacted stone during stent)
Injury to adjacent organs	No risk with stent, PCN may injure bowel/lung/spleen
Resource/availability	Stent does not require radiologist
Urine output monitoring	PCN allows monitoring of output from kidney
Ureteric access	Available after PCN, not stent

STONE TREATMENTS OVERVIEW

STONE OBSERVATION

The younger the patient, the larger the stone and the more symptomatic the stone is, the more likely that treatment will be recommended.

Staghorn calculi are not routinely recommended to undergo observation (mortality ≤ 30% due to renal causes) unless comorbidities pose higher risk during surgery.

Further consideration is occupation (e.g. airline pilot, bus or lorry driver), as such patients may have to be radiologically stone free before they are allowed to work again.

Employees should be encouraged to inform their relevant authority e.g. DVLA, Civil Aviation Authority.

Kidney Stones

The natural history of small asymptomatic kidney stones remains unclear – it remains debatable whether they should be actively treated or followed-up.

NICE advises watchful waiting can be considered for asymptomatic renal stones if:

- Stone is < 5mm
- Stone is ≥ 5mm and patient agrees to watchful waiting after risks vs. benefits discussion.

Evidence is conflicting and based mainly on single-centre observational studies, such as:

- *Glowacki et al.* – followed up 107 patients for 31 months – symptomatic event only 32%, of which half passed their stone conservatively [13]
- *Dropkin et al.* – followed up 110 patients over 3 years, finding only 24% symptomatic and 19% requiring surgical intervention. [14]

Ureteric Stones

The cardinal factors to warrant intervention are infection, intractable pain or obstruction.

NICE recommends surgical treatment/ESWL be offered to adults with ureteric stones within 48 hours of diagnosis if pain is ongoing and stone unlikely to pass.

89% of lower ureteric and 71% of upper ureteric stones < 5mm in size will pass spontaneously.

MIMIC study (covered below) found a high overall stone passage rate with conservative management.

EAU 2024 supports initial observation of patients with newly diagnosed small ureteric stones, provided active removal is not indicated (e.g. intractable pain, renal failure).

CHEMOLYSIS

Oral chemolysis requires alkalinisation of the urine with potassium citrate or sodium bicarbonate.

The urinary pH should ideally be 7.0–7.2; however, at a higher pH it may be more effective at the expense of increased risk of calcium phosphate stone formation.

Uric acid and cystine stones are potentially suitable for chemolysis.

EAU 2024 recommends patients should be taught how to self-monitor their urine pH and adjust their alkalising medication dose accordingly.

The non-palatable taste of the medication can be a limiting factor of patient compliance.

MEDICAL EXPULSIVE THERAPY

MET in the form of α-blockers (tamsulosin, terazosin, doxazosin are equally effective) remains a debated topic within urology in the treatment of ureteric stones.

MET should not be used in the infected obstructed kidney.

Patient should be counselled regarding side-effects (e.g. postural hypotension and retrograde ejaculation), that the drug use is "off-label" and evidence for MET efficacy is controversial.

EAU 2024 continues to recommend offering α-blockers as MET as one of the treatment options for distal and larger (> 5mm) ureteric stones, provided conservative management is safe.

NICE states that MET should be considered in distal ureteric stones < 10mm in size.

> **KEY PAPER** | SUSPEND Trial (2015) [15]

- Multi-centre, randomised placebo-controlled UK-based trial published in the *Lancet*.
- Recruited > 1,000 patients with CT-proven single ureteric stone to (tamsulosin) vs. (placebo) vs. (nifedipine) (1:1:1).
- Primary outcome was need for treatment/intervention within 4 weeks.
- No difference was found between groups (i.e. often quoted as evidence against MET).
- Study limitations include end-point (did not prove that the stone had indeed passed) and that the majority of stones were < 5mm and thus would have passed anyway.

> **KEY PAPER** | MIMIC Study (2019) [16]

- Multi-centre, retrospective study across 71 centres in 4 countries.
- > 4,000 patients with acute colic and CT-proven single ureteric stone were reviewed to evaluate for spontaneous stone passage.
- > 2,500 were discharged with conservative management (overall passage rate 74%).
- Study did not find any benefit of MET.

> **VIVA** | Questions about whether you would use MET or not are common in the FRCS (Urol) viva as they require a discussion and review of the evidence. I strongly recommend you familiarise yourself with the above two papers and read them fully, and are able to discuss the pros and cons of MET.

EXTRA-CORPOREAL SHOCKWAVE LITHOTRIPSY (ESWL)

Three types of ESWL are available (electrohydraulic, electromagnetic and piezoelectric) – these are covered in more detail in Chapter 6, "Urological Imaging & Principles of Urological Technology".

XR and/or US can be used to locate the stone for ESWL treatment.

The most difficult stones to fragment with ESWL are calcium oxalate monohydrate.

Contraindications to undergoing ESWL include:

- Pregnancy (potential effects to foetus)
- Uncontrolled bleeding diatheses
- Active UTI
- Skeletal malformations/obesity/aneurysm in vicinity of stone
- Anatomical obstruction distal to the stone.

Side-effects of ESWL include:

- Visible haematuria, pain, urinary tract infection
- Failure of treatment or need for further sessions
- *Steinstrasse* obstruction.

NICE does not recommend routine stenting prior to ESWL as it does not improve SFR or lower number of auxiliary treatments.

NICE suggests consider MET as adjunctive therapy in adults having ESWL for ureteric stones < 10mm.

EAU 2024 recommends routine analgesia as it is beneficial because it limits pain-induced movements.

EAU 2024 recommends routine antibiotic prophylaxis only in case of ureteric stent in situ, infected stones and/or bacteriuria.

Patients with pacemaker and ICD can be treated with ESWL with caution.

There is no strong evidence to suggest causal link between ESWL and diabetes or hypertension.

Optimal shockwave frequency is 1–1.5Hz; however, there is no consensus on maximum number of shockwaves per session.

Efficacy of ESWL depends on:

1. Stone size: more effective for stones < 1cm diameter
2. Stone location: less effective in lower pole stones and/or in calyceal diverticulum
3. Stone composition: less effective in cystine or calcium oxalate monohydrate stones
4. Best practice: user experience, with optimised acoustic coupling gel, frequency of 1–1.5Hz
5. Anatomical: increasing skin-to-stone distance reduces efficacy (> 10cm), narrow infundibulum (< 5mm) or steep infundibular-pelvic angle.

ESWL can be used as upfront treatment for non-infected ureteric stones that are unlikely to pass and need intervention (see TISU trial below).

| KEY PAPER | TISU Trial (2021) [17]

- Multi-centre, randomised UK-based trial published which aimed to evaluate non-inferiority of upfront ≤ 2 ESWL sessions vs. URS as initial treatment for ureteric stones.
- > 600 patients randomised with a CT-proven single ureteric stone needing intervention.
- (1:1) to (ESWL) vs. (URS), primary outcome as need of further intervention to clear stone.
- Found 22% of ESWL vs. 10% of URS needed further intervention (ARR 11.7%), which was inside the 20% threshold the authors set for demonstrating non-inferiority.

URETEROSCOPY

Rigid URS scopes have tip diameters 7–10Fr (working channel 3.4Fr) and can be used for the entire ureter, and should always be used alongside a safety wire.

Flexible URS scopes are smaller (distal tip < 9Fr) and accommodate working channel 3.6Fr.

Ho:YAG LASER is the most effective LASER to treat stones (solid-state pulsed LASER) in URS.

Ho:YAG has a favourable safety profile due to controlled shallow penetration depth and water absorption characteristics (meaning reduction of energy reaching non-target tissue).

LASER energy is delivered down a fibre with diameter 200–360µm.

Smaller fibres (e.g. 200µm) allow greater flexibility and preferable to use for kidney stones.

The zone of thermal injury is limited to 0.5–1mm from the LASER tip.

No stone can withstand the heat generated from Ho:YAG LASER; however, harder stones will take longer to fragment/dust.

URS + LASER are most suited for stones < 2cm diameter (reducing efficacy as stone burden increases).

The following are a list of potential *indications* to undergo primary elective URS:

- Failed ESWL or hard stones (high HU on CT KUB)
- ESWL unlikely to be successful (e.g. larger lower pole stone)
- Stone in calyceal diverticulum or infundibulum (may require incising)
- Obesity, horseshoe kidney, patient preference, pregnancy.

LASER Settings

There are 3 parameters which are important to consider when fragmenting stones:

- *Frequency* – increasing (30–50Hz) aids dusting (low Hz yields larger fragments)
- *Energy* – low J (0.3–0.6J) favours dusting, high energy increases risk of retropulsion
- *Pulse width/duration* – longer pulse modes (800µs) result in less retropulsion.

The frequency multiplied by the energy gives the power of the LASER.

Access Sheaths

Hydrophilic-coated ureteral access sheaths (inner diameter ≥ 9F) can be inserted via guidewire placing the sheath tip in the proximal ureter.

Allows easy multiple access to upper tract, improves intra-operative vision due to continuous irrigation and reduces operative time.

Access-sheath insertion may increase the risk of ureteral injury (risk reduced in pre-stented systems).

Stenting after URS

Routine stenting prior to URS is not indicated – although when present (e.g. prior emergency insertion) stenting facilitates future URS, improves SFR and reduces intra-operative complications.

Routine stenting after uncomplicated URS is not indicated and may be associated with higher post-operative morbidity (EAU 2024 and NICE).

Consider overnight placement of ureteric catheter instead with similar benefits.

EAU 2024 recommends stent insertion after URS be considered in the following circumstances: [10]

- Ureteric trauma/perforation during the procedure
- Residual stone fragments > 2mm within ureter
- Bleeding
- URS during pregnancy
- Impacted stone cases/prolonged procedures.

EAU 2024 recommends offering MET to patients with stent-related symptoms after URS.

PERCUTANEOUS NEPHROLITHOTOMY

PCNL remains standard procedure for large renal calculi.

Standard access tracts are 24–30Fr; however, smaller outer diameter sheaths are being used e.g. mini-PCNL 14–20Fr, ultra-mini PCNL 11–13Fr, micro-PCNL < 11Fr.

Collecting system is first inflated via fluid from cystoscopically inserted ureteric catheter, followed by percutaneous needle into calyx, guidewire insertion and sequential tract dilatation.

CT imaging prior to surgery is essential to provide information regarding interposition of organs.

Lower pole access is generally favoured in emergency setting (e.g. nephrostomy insertion).

Upper pole access is favoured for PCNL as it provides straight line to PUJ and access to all calyces.

The following are a list of potential *indications* to undergo PCNL:

- Obstruction distal to stone location (i.e. cannot use ESWL)
- Patient preference for greatest chance of clearance in single treatment session
- Failed ESWL/URS
- Stone size (> 3cm/staghorn, or renal pelvis > 2cm or lower pole stone > 1cm).

Contraindications to undergoing PCNL include:

- Uncorrected bleeding disorder
- Pregnancy, sepsis and/or poor kidney function
- Confirmed or potential malignant renal tumour.

Common side-effects of PCNL include:

- Pain, bleeding, infection/sepsis
- Multiple puncture sites for access/failure to clear stones
- Major bleeding requiring emergency embolisation ($\leq$ 1%)
- Injury to bowel/liver/lung
- Major bleeding requiring nephrectomy (< 0.1%).

Colonic Injury in PCNL

Signs of colonic injury may be mild and late, due to retro-peritoneal location and containment.

A ureteric stent should be placed to decompress system, withdraw nephrostomy from intra-renal position to intra-colonic thus serving as colostomy tube (keep > 7 days).

Perform nephrostogram prior to tube removal to ensure no colon to kidney communication.

Supine vs. Prone PCNL

EAU 2024 does not express a preference between supine or prone positions as they are equally safe, the SFR are comparable and operative time similar. [10]

Table 6 – Comparison of supine vs. prone PCNL techniques

Advantage of Supine PCNL	Advantage of Prone PCNL
Patient positioning faster and less risk of injury	Wider area / more options for puncture
Reduced anaesthetic / cardiovascular complications	May reduce risk of visceral organ damage
Simultaneous retrograde access to collect system	Greater manipulation of nephroscope

Tubeless PCNL

Tubeless PCNL is performed without a PCN, *totally tubeless* PCNL without PCN or ureteric stent.

EAU 2024 recommends tubeless or totally tubeless PCNL for uncomplicated cases. [10]

Totally tubeless PCNL is associated with shorter in-patient hospital stays.

Routine nephrostomy tube placement will depend on various factors including:

- Likelihood of second-look procedure/large residual stones
- Single kidney
- Significant intra-operative blood loss
- Ureteral obstruction
- Urine extravasation/bacteriuria/infection stones.

VIVA If asked in your FRCS (Urol) viva about which intervention you would choose for a given ureteric or kidney stone in a non-emergency scenario, categorise the stone based on size and location and then refer to the relevant NICE or EAU treatment algorithm per category:

- NICE categorises kidney stones as < 10mm, 10–20mm, > 20mm
- NICE categorises ureteric stones as < 10mm, 10–20mm
- EAU further subdivides kidney stones into lower and non-lower pole
- EAU further subdivides ureteric stones into proximal and distal.

LOWER POLE CALCULI

BROAD PRINCIPLES

Stratified by stone size, lower pole stones fair worse than other sites.

This is likely due to poor clearance of fragments from the dependent lower pole, as the disintegration efficacy of ESWL is otherwise no different to stones elsewhere in the kidney.

Obtuse angles are likely to be more favourable for ESWL clearance than acute angles.

Anatomical factors which may further limit efficacy of ESWL for treating lower pole stones: [18–19]

- Steep infundibulo-pelvic angle
- Long calyx (> 10mm)
- Narrow infundibulum (< 5mm)
- Long skin-to-stone distance (> 10cm).

If there are negative predictors for ESWL, then PCNL or URS are reasonable alternatives.

MANAGEMENT

Not all lower pole stones require treatment and many can be observed.

EAU 2024 indications for active stone removal for kidney stones include: [10]

- Stone growth
- Symptomatic stones (pain, infection, haematuria)
- Stones causing obstruction
- Patient preference/occupation/comorbidity.

ESWL, PCNL or FURS are available options for lower pole stones that require treatment.

Figure 2 – EAU 2024 lower pole stone treatment algorithm [10]

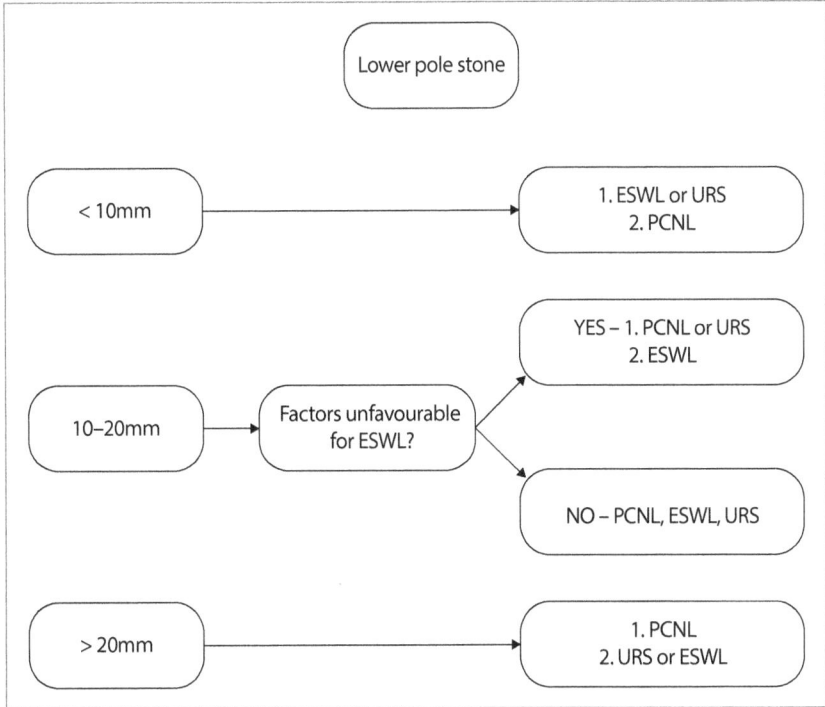

COMPARING TREATMENTS

KEY PAPER | Lower Pole I [20]

- Prospective randomised multi-centre trial comparing PCNL (128) vs. ESWL (128) for lower pole stones < 30mm, published in 2001.
- SFR at 3 months were 95% (PCNL) vs. 37% (ESWL).
- Complication rates were 23% (PCNL) vs. 13% (ESWL).
- Re-treatment rates were 11% (PCNL) vs. 31% (ESWL).

Main drawback of study was lack of comparison with FURS (addressed in Lower Pole Study II).

| **KEY PAPER** | Lower Pole II [21] |

- Prospective, randomised, multi-centre trial published in 2005.
- 78 patients with isolated ≤ 10mm lower pole stones randomised to ESWL vs. URS.
- No statistically significant difference in SFR was found (although URS was 15% better).
- Greater operative time and complications were noted in URS group.

Currently, the PCNL, FURS and ESWL study (*PUrE*) is underway in the UK to compare cost and clinical effectiveness of the different modalities of treatment. Results due.

URETERIC CALCULI

DIAGNOSTIC EVALUATION

Perform urinalysis to evaluate for NVH, send bloods for FBC, UE, CRP and serum calcium/uric acid.

Always undertake a pregnancy test in women with abdominal pain of child-bearing age.

Obtain urgent imaging.

> **VIVA** Always keep an open mind in your FRCS (Urol) viva. You may be presented with a sick-patient scenario who has classical loin-to-groin pain; it may be tempting to run with the assumption it is a stone-related pathology. However, the underlying issue could be surgical, for example, and completely unrelated; therefore screen for such pathology in your history taking and let the examiners know you are adopting a broad approach to the patient.

MANAGEMENT

Patient should be resuscitated in a systematic Airway-to-Exposure manner, ensuring that the Sepsis-6 bundle has been completed.

Provide analgesia early (first-line NSAIDs), consider IV paracetamol.

Any documented fever should be taken very seriously and treated as sepsis due to infected obstructed kidney until proven otherwise.

Observation

Stone size is the main determinant of the success of conservative management.

Estimated that spontaneous stone passage rates ≤ 95% of ureteric stones ≤ 4mm in size.

Observation is a reasonable strategy for those who do not develop complications (infection, intractable pain, renal impairment) or have no social reasons to warrant intervention.

Larger stones are unlikely to pass and should not routinely undergo a period of observation.

Irreversible kidney damage may occur within 2–4 weeks if ureteric stone is completely obstructing.

Medical Expulsive Therapy

Please consult the relevant section in "Stone Treatments Overview".

MET is most likely to be beneficial in distal ureteric stones > 5mm in size.

Emergency Drainage

Please consult the relevant section in "Stones: Broad Principles".

EAU 2024 recommends PCN or stenting are both suitable options in the emergency context: [10]

- Key factor in choice is earliest intervention
- Urine should be collected directly from the obstructed kidney when drained.

ESWL vs. URS

Treatment guidelines factor ureteric stone patients as index – adult, non-pregnant, normal contra-lateral kidney, no comorbidities, no kidney stones, single ureteric stone.

NICE guidelines for surgical treatment of ureteric stones:

- < 10mm: offer ESWL, consider URS (e.g. contraindications to ESWL, ESWL failed)
- > 10mm: offer URS, consider ESWL if local facilities allow prompt access.

EAU 2024 surgical treatment of ureteric stones further subdivides ureter into proximal and distal:

- Proximal < 10mm: offer URS or ESWL
- Proximal > 10mm: first choice URS, second choice ESWL
- Distal < 10mm: offer URS or ESWL
- Distal > 10mm: first choice URS, second choice ESWL.

Inform patients that URS has better chance of achieving stone-free status with single intervention.

Inform patients that URS has higher complication rates compared to ESWL.

Many departments will not have 24-hour access to ESWL machine/technicians and therefore resource availability will impact management decisions.

ESWL is unlikely to be successful in severely obese patients and should not be considered first choice.

PHYSIOLOGY OF UPPER-TRACT OBSTRUCTION

Animal experiments on the physiological response to complete ureteral occlusion yielded findings regarding the kidney's compensatory mechanisms.

Phase I (0–90 minutes):

- Pre-glomerular vasodilatation increases renal blood flow in response to ureteral pressure rise.
- Compensatory mechanism to increase capillary hydrostatic pressure/GFR.

Phase II (90 minutes – 5 hours)

- Reduction in renal blood flow despite continued rise in ureteral pressure, due to post-glomerular vasoconstriction (further attempt by kidney to maintain GFR).

Phase III (> 5 hours)

- Fall in both renal blood flow and ureteral pressure due to pre-glomerular vasoconstriction (mediated by eicosanoids, renin, angiotensin II).

STAGHORN CALCULI

EPIDEMIOLOGY

Staghorn calculi are result of rUTI and are thus more common in women, renal tract anomalies, SCI patients, neurogenic bladder or ileal diversion. [22]

PATHOLOGY

Staghorn calculi are composed of struvite (pure struvite is magnesium ammonium phosphate).

Triple phosphate is a term often used interchangeably with struvite, although strictly speaking pure struvite does not contain calcium, whilst triple phosphate is calcium magnesium ammonium.

Struvite accounts for ~70% of their composition and is usually mixed with calcium phosphate which will render them radio-opaque.

The following conditions must be met for struvite stones to develop:

- Alkaline urine pH > 7.2
- Ammonia in urine
- UTI with urease-producing organisms (Proteus, Klebsiella, Enterobacter) which hydrolyses urea to ammonium and CO_2.

VIVA   You may be asked in the FRCS (Urol) viva to draw on paper the equation for formation of staghorn calculi in front of the examiners – make sure you can do this confidently (Figure 3).

Figure 3 – Equation for formation of staghorn calculi

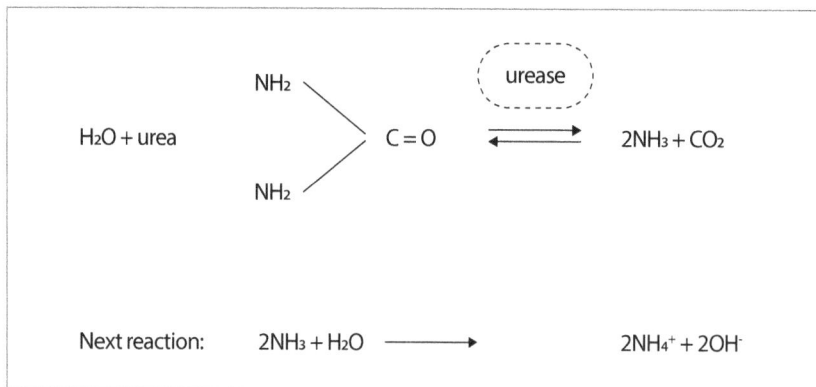

$$H_2O + urea \quad \begin{matrix} NH_2 \\ \diagup \\ C=O \\ \diagdown \\ NH_2 \end{matrix} \quad \underset{urease}{\overset{}{\rightleftharpoons}} \quad 2NH_3 + CO_2$$

Next reaction: $2NH_3 + H_2O \longrightarrow 2NH_4^+ + 2OH^-$

DIAGNOSTIC EVALUATION

Patients are deemed high risk and therefore should undergo thorough metabolic work-up.

Check urinary pH, send MSU, bloods for FBC, UE, CRP, serum calcium and uric acid.

DMSA is recommended prior to major surgical intervention, to obtain split kidney function which will ultimately determine management.

CTU is recommended to map the calyces to plan optimal puncture access to the kidney.

MANAGEMENT

Staghorn calculi should be treated surgically, provided the patient is clinically fit and the affected kidney is adequately functioning on DMSA – observation is no longer routinely recommended.

The key principles in the management of staghorn calculi are:

1. Clear the stone (PCNL/URS) and infection (antibiotics)
2. High fluid intake
3. Consider acidifying the urine.

Both NICE and EAU recommend PCNL be offered as first-choice surgical intervention for large kidney stones.

Open or laparoscopic stone removal is a valid option in rare cases where all other modalities have failed or are unlikely to be successful (EAU 2024).

Acetohydroxamic acid is a drug which competitively inhibits urease, and although it can help prevent stone recurrence its use is limited by side-effects (risk of DVT, hair loss, haemolytic anaemia).

KEY PAPER | Blandy and Singh (1976) [23]

- Article advocating a more active approach to treating staghorn calculi, in 3 parts.
- *Post-mortem* study, 9 / 8,996 post-mortems found a staghorn (and 5 / 9 died of related causes).
- *Retrospective* study of 60 observed staghorn calculi, where overall 17 / 60 died (28%), 20 / 60 had early nephrectomy and of the remaining 40, 16 developed pyonephrosis.
- *Case series* of 125 patients treated for staghorn calculi (lower mortality of 7%).

KEY PAPER | Teichman et al. (1995) [24]

- Retrospective analysis of 177 consecutive staghorn calculi over > 7 years mean follow-up.
- No patient with complete clearance died, 3% with residual fragments died and 67% of those who refused treatment died.

KEY PAPER | Deutsch and Subramonian (2016) [25]

- Prospective cohort study in single centre of 22 patients with staghorn calculi undergoing conservative management.
- Yearly review of clinical status and GFR measurement.
- Progressive renal failure (14%), disease-specific mortality (9%).
- Authors concluded that conservative management was not as unsafe as previously thought.

VIVA | You may be asked in the FRCS (Urol) viva how you would manage a staghorn calculus. This is a typical question where candidates would be expected to discuss the relevant evidence in order to achieve high marks.

STONES IN SPECIFIC GROUPS

STONES IN PREGNANCY

EPIDEMIOLOGY

Pregnant patients do not appear to be at increased risk of stone formation compared to non-pregnant females of similar child-bearing age.

Urolithiasis is estimated to affect 1 in 200 pregnancies.

Occurs most commonly in second/third trimester and is associated with pre-term labour.

PATHOPHYSIOLOGY

The overall net effect of physiological changes in pregnancy does not increase risk of stone formation.

Factors promoting stone formation in pregnancy include:

- Physiological hydronephrosis and ureteric smooth muscle dilatation (progesterone)
- Hypercalciuria (suppression of PTH)
- Increased uric acid/calcium/oxalate excretion.

These are counterbalanced by increased filtration of stone inhibitors (citrate/GAG/magnesium). [7]

Physiological hydronephrosis is more common on the right (90%) due to:

- Compression by dilated right ovarian vein
- Uterine dextro-rotation
- Protection of the left ureter by gas-filled sigmoid colon.

Treatment is not usually required for physiological hydronephrosis unless intractable pain/sepsis, in which case drainage should be performed (evaluate for obstructing stone as cause).

Physiological hydronephrosis will usually resolve within 6 weeks of delivery.

DIAGNOSTIC EVALUATION

Urinanalysis and MSU should be performed, bloods for FBC/UE/LFT/CRP.

Urgent review by obstetric team is mandatory.

Imaging

EAU 2024 recommends the following imaging modalities in pregnancy: [10]

- First line: US as preferred method
- Second line: MRI (if US equivocal, allows definition of obstruction level, view of other organs)
- Third line: low-dose CT KUB with foetal shield (avoid where possible).

US has poor sensitivity for ureteric stones (transvaginal may help with distal stones) and cannot differentiate between acute obstruction and physiological hydronephrosis of pregnancy.

MANAGEMENT

The patient should be resuscitated in a systematic Airway-to-Exposure manner ensuring the Sepsis-6 bundle has been completed when applicable.

A multi-disciplinary approach recommended with input from obstetrics, urology, radiology.

Pain Relief

Paracetamol and opioid analgesia are first line due to potential harmful effects of other drugs.

Avoid NSAIDs due to risk of closure of ductus arteriosus by blocking prostaglandin release.

Antibiotics

Antibiotic therapy should be based on available culture/sensitivity reports and local guidelines.

Prophylactic antibiotics should be considered as $\leq 50\%$ of pregnant patients with stones have concomitant infection.

Penicillins and cephalosporins are considered safe in pregnancy.

Avoid trimethoprim (folate antagonist), gentamicin (auditory/vestibular damage) and nitrofurantoin (neonatal haemolysis).

Conservative Approach

Approximately 15–30% of pregnant patients with stones will need active intervention, ≤ 80% of ureteric stones will pass spontaneously due to physiologically dilated upper tracts.

Conservative management consists of rest, hydration, analgesia, anti-emetics and observation.

Patients with sepsis, intractable pain or renal impairment are not suitable for observation.

Active Intervention

PCN is beneficial in that it avoids GA.

Nephrostomy disadvantages include psychological implications of urine bag, dislodgement, recurrent blockages requiring frequent changes (every 4 weeks).

The alternative option is retrograde ureteric stenting.

Stent disadvantages include risk of GA, encrustation due to hypercalciuria requiring regular GA changes, irritative stent symptoms.

The surgical treatment of choice is FURS (modified dorsal lithotomy); however, GA may induce pre-term labour and most would favour a delayed treatment approach.

EAU 2024 recommends non-urgent URS is best performed in the second trimester. [10]

ESWL is absolutely contraindicated.

PCNL should not be routinely offered but may be an option in select cases in experienced hands.

STONES IN CHILDREN

Children with urinary stones are considered high-risk stone formers, and therefore a thorough diagnostic work-up should be undertaken.

Common non-metabolic aetiological causes include VUR, PUJO and neurogenic bladder.

< 1% of urinary stones occur in patients aged < 18 years.

Premature children are at much higher risk (increased oxalate excretion).

Hypercalciuria is the most common metabolic abnormality identified in children with calculi, and hyperoxaluria is commonly found in the context of CF. [26]

Imaging

Obtaining clear imaging in children may be challenging; always adopt the ALARA approach for radiation (As Low As Reasonably Achievable).

US with a full bladder is primary imaging technique in children (sensitivity < 60%).

If US inconclusive, consider low-dose CT KUB as alternative.

Treatment Options

MET may reduce stone-expulsion times and decrease pain episodes and the expense of more side-effects; however, evidence as to its efficacy is limited.

ESWL indications are similar to those for adults:

- Potential concern regarding safety of ESWL on immature kidneys and surrounding organs
- General anaesthetic may be necessary, particularly in young children
- Children can pass fragments more easily.

ESWL is recommended by EAU 2024 as:

- First choice for single ureteric stones < 10mm and renal stones < 20mm.

PCNL indications similar to those for adults, as is the rationale for tubeless approach.

PCNL is recommended by EAU 2024 as:

- First choice for renal stones > 20mm.

URS indications similar to those for adults, and is recommended by EAU 2024 as feasible option for:

- Ureteric stones not amenable to ESWL
- Renal stones < 20mm.

STONES IN TRANSPLANT KIDNEYS

Transplant patients rely on their solitary kidney for renal function, and they are at greater risk of sepsis due to immunosuppression.

Treatment must therefore promote immediate drainage.

Hyperfiltration, RTA and raised serum calcium (tertiary PTH) are stone formation risk factors.

Treatment Options

URS can be challenging due to anterior location of implanted ureter into the bladder.

ESWL is safe but stone-localisation is difficult and SFR are poor.

EAU 2024 recommends that all options (ESWL, URS, PCNL) can be potentially offered to transplant kidney patients, but selecting the appropriate technique can be difficult.

CYSTINURIA

EPIDEMIOLOGY

Cystine stones account for 1% of adult stones and 6–8% of stones in children.

Peak incidence of stone formation is in second-to-third decade of life.

All cystine stone formers are deemed at high risk of recurrence.

Males and females are equally affected.

PATHOPHYSIOLOGY

Autosomal recessive pattern of inheritance leading to inborn error of metabolism. [27]

Patients can have homo- or heterozygous genotype; however, the phenotype is the same.

Cystinuria is an inherited kidney and intestinal trans-epithelial transport defect for the amino acids cystine, ornithine, lysine and arginine (COLA).

Features reduced proximal tubular reabsorption of the COLA amino acids.

There is excessive secretion of COLA in the urine; however, only cystine is poorly soluble and so only cystine stones are formed.

Cystinuria patients often excrete > 1g of cystine a day (well above solubility of cystine).

Cystine solubility is low in acidic urine (hence the treatment strategy of alkalinising the urine) and will crystallise spontaneously in normal physiological urinary pH range.

Cystine crystals are hexagonal shaped.

Crystals are visible in only 25% of urine specimens, and therefore confirmation of diagnosis should be via 24-hour urine collection studies.

DIAGNOSTIC EVALUATION

Stone analysis is the optimal way to establish the diagnosis of cystinuria.

If stone sample is not available, undertake 24-hour collection to detect crystals and measure urinary cystine levels, which can also help establish homo- vs. heterozygotes.

Brand's Test [7]

Also known as cyanide-nitroprusside test.

Cyanide converts cystine to cysteine, which binds to nitroprusside causing a purple hue within minutes if cystine level > 75mg/L.

Over 24-hour collection test, homozygotes (> 600mg/day) and heterozygotes (200–400mg/day).

MANAGEMENT

Surgical care is similar to that of patients with other types of stone, except cystine stones are more resistant to ESWL which may limit efficacy.

Medical care is multifaceted and focuses on stone prevention:

- *High fluid intake*, aiming for > 4L/day
- *Urine alkalinisation*, aiming for pH > 7.5 (e.g. sodium bicarbonate, potassium citrate)

- *Oral chelators* bind to cystine increasing solubility e.g. tiopronin/α-mercaptopropionylglycine (α-MPG)
- *Captopril*, a first-line ACEi which also binds to cystine to form more soluble complex.

α-MPG has similar efficacy to D-penicillamine (which binds to cysteine) in reducing urinary cystine but is far less toxic.

STONES IN HORSESHOE KIDNEYS

The prevalence of horseshoe kidneys is 1 in 400.

Due to abnormal medial fusion of metanephric blastema causing failure of ascent (by inferior mesenteric artery) and kidney rotation.

Horseshoe kidneys are more caudal in position compared to normal kidneys.

The renal pelvis lies anterior to the calyces (all calyces are lateral to renal pelvis in normal kidney) and the calyces face posteriorly and caudally.

MANAGEMENT

ESWL

Visualisation may be challenging due to overlying bowel gas and/or bony landmarks.

ESWL can be successful; however, fragment drainage can be impaired by high insertion of ureter onto renal pelvis and relative urinary stasis.

URS

URS is a treatment option; however, likely need for flexible scope due to tortuous ureteric anatomy.

High SFR are achievable – though not matching those obtained in normal kidneys.

PCNL

Large stones > 2cm or in cases of failed ESWL/URS, then PCNL should be considered.

Tract difficulties include greater length and more medial location (higher risk of colonic injury).

Usual point of access in horseshoe kidneys is the upper pole posterior calyx.

STONES IN CALCYCEAL DIVERTICULAE

A calyceal diverticulum is a non-secretory urothelial-lined compartment in (often very narrow) communication with the renal collection system.

Rationale for treatment vs. observation are the same.

ESWL has low SFR due to poor drainage of fragments through the narrow communication point.

URS can be beneficial as it occasionally allows simultaneous incision of the diverticular neck.

PCNL is superior at obliterating the diverticulum and achieving greater SFR.

STONES IN RENAL TUBULAR ACIDOSIS

RTA is a defect of renal tubular H+ excretion – impairing ability to acidify urine (pH > 5.8)

The reduced ions will reduce bicarbonate reabsorption, promoting chloride reabsorption which leads to hyperchloraemic metabolic acidosis.

This serum parameter will promote resorption of bone apatite to raise serum calcium.

Hypercalciuria ensues, which further promotes stone formation in the alkaline environment.

Confirmation of diagnosis is via ammonium chloride loading test.

The most appropriate treatment is potassium alkali (potassium citrate) as compared to sodium alkali it reduces urinary calcium (sodium alkali may increase calcium stone formation).

Type 1/Distal RTA

Distal tubule cannot maintain proton gradient between blood and tubular fluid.

70% of such patients have stones (calcium phosphate/brushite) (and often nephrocalcinosis).

Type 2/Proximal RTA

Impaired bicarbonate reabsorption in proximal tubule, increasing urinary citrate (protects against stones) and thus not a relevant condition in stone formers.

BLADDER CALCULI

EPIDEMIOLOGY

Bladder stones are more common in men and in the elderly.

More common in developing countries due to dehydration, chronic diarrhoea and dietary deficiencies.

Bladder stones are seen in ≤ 5% of those undergoing BOO surgery, ≤ 67% of SCI patients and ~2% of patients with urinary catheters.

PATHOPHYSIOLOGY

Bladder stones can be categorised as:

- *Primary*, occurring in the absence of other urinary tract abnormalities
- *Secondary*, occurring in the presence of urinary tract abnormalities (e.g. BOO, foreign bodies)
- *Migratory*, those that have passed from the upper urinary tract.

Metabolic abnormalities predisposing patients to form secondary bladder stones are poorly understood.

Studies of bladder stone analysis show varied distributions of composition, suggesting multiple metabolic factors are likely to be contributing.

Low urine volume/dehydration is the most consistently noted abnormality.

BOO is the most common predisposing factor for bladder stone formation in adults.

DIAGNOSTIC EVALUATION

Common symptoms include VH, rUTI, frequency and dysuria, and these may be exacerbated by sudden movement (e.g. rising to stand).

10% are diagnosed incidentally on imaging.

Perform urinalysis, send MSU and measure urinary pH, bloods for FBC, UE, serum calcium and uric acid.

Examine external genitalia, perform DRE and peripheral neurological examination, offer uroflowmetry with PVR assessment.

Imaging

US is a good imaging modality to detect bladder stones (sensitivity ≤ 83%).

CT KUB is more sensitive, however, and has the benefit of being able to accurately evaluate for upper-tract urolithiasis.

No study compares cystoscopy and CT for diagnosis of bladder stones.

MANAGEMENT

Migratory small stones are typically treated conservatively with the expectation that these will pass.

Primary and secondary stones are usually symptomatic and require treatment.

Medical treatment (chemolysis) is not routinely employed and evidence in its support is weak.

Trans-urethral Cystolithotripsy

Trans-urethral cystolithotripsy should be offered as first choice where possible (EAU 2024).

Mechanical, pneumatic and LASER are equivalent lithotripsy modalities for use in endoscopic bladder stone treatment – choice will depend on surgeon preference and local resources.

Concomitant BOO surgery should be considered, but not imperative at time of bladder stone removal.

Patients rendered stone-free from surgery may subsequently be medically managed for BPH without the need for BOO surgery.

Concomitant BOO surgery may be appropriate in patients with voiding LUTS refractory to medical management and/or UDS proven obstruction, recurrent urinary retention.

Complication rates for trans-urethral cystolithotripsy are similar if BOO surgery is performed at same time.

Suprapubic Cystolithotomy

Open bladder stone extraction may be offered as an option for very large stones (EAU 2024).

Associated with increased length of in-patient stay compared to trans-urethral cystolithotripsy.

Follow-up

Follow-up strategy will be tailored to individual patient circumstances.

Patients with bladder stones in the context of BOO may require follow-up uroflowmetry with PVR or UDS (if not previously performed).

Routine follow-up cystoscopy is not currently recommended.

URINARY TRACT INFECTIONS: BROAD PRINCIPLES

TERMINOLOGY

UTI – bacterial invasion of the urothelium resulting in an inflammatory response

Bacteriuria – presence of bacteria in the urine (bacteriuria without pyuria suggests colonisation)

Pyuria – presence of white blood cells in urine

Sterile pyuria – presence of white blood cells in urine with bacteriuria (e.g. TB, CIS, interstitial cystitis)

Cystitis – syndrome of dysuria, frequency, urgency with or without suprapubic pain

Acute pyelonephritis – syndrome comprising of flank pain, nausea/vomiting, fever > 38°C

Chronic pyelonephritis – radiological diagnosis describing scarred, shrunken kidney which may or may not have resulted from recurrent infections

Uncomplicated UTI – occurring in a patient with structurally and functionally normal urinary tract

Complicated UTI – in presence of underlying anatomical or functional abnormality also including:

- All men
- Pregnant women
- Indwelling catheters or stents, immuno-compromised, renal disease
- Hospital-acquired infections

Isolated UTI – occurs > 6 months after the previous UTI

Recurrent UTI – ≥ 2 UTI in 6 months or ≥ 3 UTI in 12 months (EAU and NICE):

- *Persistent* – rUTI caused by same organism
- *Re-infection* – episodes of UTI caused by different organisms

Unresolved infection – one that has not responded to treatment (e.g. antimicrobial resistance)

Pathogenicity – the ability of an organism to cause disease

Virulence – degree of pathogenicity

Opportunistic infections – caused by non-pathogens (commensals) due to weakened host defence

Bacteriostatic – agent which stops bacteria reproducing whilst not necessarily killing them (bactericidal agents kill bacteria)

URINE TESTING

There are different possible colours of urine with listed causes:

- Cloudy: phosphaturia (commonest cause), pyuria
- Red: haematuria, myo-/haemoglobinuria, rifampicin, chronic lead/ mercury poisoning
- Orange: dehydration, sulfasalazine
- Green/blue: biliverdin, methylene blue, amitriptyline
- Brown/black: urobilinogen, porphyria, metronidazole, nitrofurantoin, laxatives, melanin.

Most accurate urine specimen for culture is suprapubic aspirate (avoids introducing urethral bacteria).

URINE DIPSTICK TEST

Blood

Orthotolidine (a peroxidase substrate) on dipstick comes into contact with haemoglobin (contains peroxidase activity) leading to oxidation reaction and cell lysis on strip. [28]

Same reaction occurs with myo- and haemoglobinuria.

The resulting colour change on strip is blue.

Urinalysis for non-visible haematuria may be misleading due to:

- False positives – (oxidising agents) exercise, dehydration, menstrual blood
- False negatives – (reducing agents) vitamin C.

Leucocytes

Neutrophils (in infected urine) produce leucocyte esterase.

Leucocyte esterase causes hydrolysis of substrate on strip to produce indoxyl, which oxidises diazonium salt chromogen on strip to produce colour change violet.

Urinalysis for leucocytes may be misleading due to:

- False positives – specimen contamination e.g. vaginal discharge
- False negatives – old specimen (leucocyte lysis), dehydration, vitamin C, urobilinogen.

Sensitivity for UTI is 70–95% (not all patients with bacteriuria have pyuria).

Nitrites

Most Gram-negative bacteria (i.e. most common uropathogens) convert nitrates (present in urine) to nitrites (not usually present in urine).

Nitrites react with aromatic amine on dipstick to produce colour change pink.

Griess reaction (detects presence of nitrite ion in solution) takes 4 hours.

Urinalysis for nitrites may be misleading due to:

- False positives – contamination
- False negatives – Gram-negative bacteria (e.g. Pseudomonas), urine in bladder < 4 hours.

High specificity for UTI (90–100%); however, lower sensitivity than leucocytes (35–85%).

Regarding urinalysis for UTI, NICE 2024 proposes:

- If dipstick is positive for nitrite or leucocyte and RBC, then UTI is likely
- If dipstick is negative for all nitrite, leucocyte and RBC, then UTI is unlikely.

pH

Average urinary pH is 5.5–6.5.

Alkaline pH > 7.5 in context of UTI suggests presence of stones.

Certain organisms (e.g. Proteus, Klebsiella, Pseudomonas) produce urease:

- Catalyses urea -> CO_2 + ammonia (ammonia raises urinary pH)
- Alkalinity causes precipitation of calcium magnesium ammonium phosphate (staghorn).

Proteins

≤ 150mg of protein is normally excreted in urine daily – any excess of this is termed proteinuria.

Dipstick contains tetrabromophenol which turns blue with albumin (> 20mg/dL).

Urinalysis for nitrites may be misleading due to:

- False negatives – dilute urine, high pH, non-albumin proteinuria (e.g. Bence-Jones in myeloma).

Glucose

In normal conditions almost all glucose should be reabsorbed at proximal convoluted tubule, unless renal reabsorption threshold is exceeded (glucose > 180mg/dL).

Glycosuria may occur after sugar-rich meal or in diabetic patients.

Double oxidation of glucose results in colour change; this is specific to glucose and not other sugars.

Specific Gravity

Measure of density of the substances dissolved in urine; depends on mass of dissolved particles.

The test strip only measures cation concentration.

Will be raised in dehydration and diuretics, reduced in overhydration or diabetes insipidus.

MIDSTREAM URINE CULTURE

For the following patients, the ideal preparation of a MSU sample involves:

- Circumcised men – no preparation (void > 100mL and then collect MSU)
- Uncircumcised men – retract foreskin, wash glans with soap, provide sample as above
- Women – retract labia, clean peri-urethral area with soap, provide sample as above.

MSU should preferably be analysed within hours, alternatively refrigerate and analyse within 24 hours.

For microscopy, 5–10mL of sample is centrifuged for 5 minutes to collect sediment.

For culture, 0.1mL is delivered onto each half of split-agar plate and cultured overnight:

- One half has blood-agar for Gram-positive organisms
- One half has eosin-methylene blue for Gram-negative organisms.

The number of CFU are then estimated.

Asymptomatic bacteriuria in women is defined as ≥ 10cfu/mL on MSU without any symptoms. [29]

GRAM STAINING

Staining method to distinguish bacterial species into 2 groups: Gram positive/negative.

Gram staining differentiates bacteria by chemical properties of cell wall by detecting peptidoglycan.

The Gram stain procedure is carried out as follows:

- Bacterial smear is stained on slide with crystal violet for 1 minute
- Gram's iodine added for 1 minute and then poured off and slide is washed with acetone
- Slide is then washed with water and safranin counterstain.

The cell wall containing peptidoglycan will remain violet colour (i.e. Gram positive). [28]

BACTERIAL VIRULENCE VS. HOST DEFENCE

The characteristics of uropathogens allowing them to colonise a host are *bacterial virulence factors*.

These can be directed against external agents e.g. antimicrobial resistance, can be chromosomal inherited, arise from mutations or be independent from chromosomes via plasmids

Alternatively, factors directed against the host:

- Toxin production, enzyme production (e.g. urease), anti-humoral substance production
- Adherence mechanisms – bacteria adhere to urothelial epithelium and initiate UTI by expressing proteins called *adhesins* on their cell surface (can be in form of fimbrae/pili or may be afimbrial).

E.coli has well-known pili facilitating adherence including:

- *Type 1*, associated with cystitis (mannose sensitive) (produced by all strains of E.coli)
- *P-pili*, associated with > 90% cases of pyelonephritis (mannose resistant)
- *S-pili*, associated with ascending UTI, sepsis, meningitis.

Conversely a number of host defence mechanisms exist to fight against the development of UTI:

- Antegrade flow of urine
- Exfoliation of urothelial cells
- Presence of intact GAG-layer
- Commensal flora of vagina (lactobacilli lower pH by converting glycogen to lactic acid)
- Tamm–Horsfall protein (made by loop of Henle) binds type-1 E.coli pili to prevent adherence.

ANTIBIOTICS

Antibiotic stewardship is a wider healthcare approach to promoting and monitoring judicious use of antimicrobials to safeguard their future effectiveness. [30]

The methods of action of common antibiotics are listed in Table 7.

Antibiotic prophylaxis for surgery should be given ≤ 30 minutes prior to start of the procedure.

Table 7 – Mechanism of actions of common antibiotics used in urinary tract infections [28]

Antibiotic	Action	Mechanism
Quinolones (e.g. ciprofloxacin)	Bacteriostatic	Prevent DNA replication by inhibiting DNA gyrase
Macrolides (e.g. erythromycin)	Bacteriostatic	Inhibit protein synthesis
Tetracyclines (e.g. doxycycline)	Bacteriostatic	Inhibit protein synthesis
Trimethoprim	Bacteriostatic	Prevent DNA replication by inhibiting dihydrofolate reductase
Penicillins (e.g. co-amoxiclav)	Bactericidal	Interfere with bacterial wall synthesis
Cephalosporins (e.g. cefalexin)	Bactericidal	Interfere with bacterial wall synthesis
Aminoglycosides (e.g. gentamicin)	Bactericidal	Inhibit protein synthesis
Nitrofurantoin	Bactericidal	Damages bacterial DNA

RECURRENT URINARY TRACT INFECTIONS

DEFINITIONS

rUTI is defined as > 2 UTI in 6 months, or ≥ 3 within 12 months.

These can be complicated or uncomplicated (and lower and upper tract); however, repeated upper tract infection should prompt consideration of complicated aetiology.

Bacterial persistence leads to recurrence within days/weeks usually by same organism.

Re-infection usually occurs after prolonged interval and often caused by different organism.

RISK FACTORS

Men with re-infection are likely to have BOO (urine is sterile in between episodes) and should be investigated with uroflowmetry, PVR and flexible cystoscopy.

In women with re-infection, functional/anatomical abnormality is unlikely; however, vaginal mucosal receptivity for uropathogen is increased predisposing them to rUTI.

Some women who suffer with rUTI may be inherently more susceptible due to their increased epithelial cell receptivity for uropathogens.

ABO blood-group antigen secretory status refers to ability of individual to secrete blood-group antigens, which is part of innate immunity against infectious disease.

The trait of increased susceptibility to UTI is associated with HLA-A3 phenotype, Lewis blood-group status (Le a-b-) and (Le a+b-), P blood-group secretors and ABO non-secretors.

Table 8 – Age-related risk factors for rUTI in women [28]

Young and Pre-menopausal	Post-menopausal and Elderly
Sexual intercourse (promote colonisation)	Urinary incontinence
Use of spermicide (promote colonisation)	Atrophic vaginitis (low oestrogen) (promote colonisation)
New sexual partner	Increased PVR volume
Mother with history of UTI	History of UTI before menopause
History of UTI in childhood	Cystocoele
Blood-group antigen secretory status	Blood-group antigen secretory status

DIAGNOSTIC EVALUATION

Patient *history* should enquire regarding the following:

- Distinguish between isolated or rUTI, and upper vs. lower tract
- Sexual history and relevant association of UTI
- Past urological history/factors suggesting UTI may be complicated
- Fluid intake, use of antibiotics, wiping patterns
- Pregnancy status and use of oral contraceptive
- Past medical history/drugs/immuno-compromised status.

Patient *examination* (with chaperone present) should evaluate for:

- Any underlying anatomical predisposing factors (e.g. palpable kidney or bladder)
- Female genitalia evidence of cystocoele, tissue oestrogenisation, prolapse, atrophic vaginitis.

Urinalysis should be performed followed by MSU formal culture and sensitivities.

Blood tests to include FBC, UE, CRP, HBA1c.

Imaging may include US KUB with PVR assessment, or CT KUB to evaluate for stones.

MANAGEMENT

In an acute UTI scenario, antimicrobial therapy is recommended because clinical success is more likely compared with placebo.

The choice of antibiotic is guided by local guidelines, allergies, sensitivities and pregnancy status.

Nitrofurantoin 100mg (PO) BD or trimethoprim 200mg (PO) BD are common first-line choices.

PREVENTION

Address any reversible factors if detected on lifestyle choices/examination/blood tests/imaging.

If investigations revealed no reversible factors, it is challenging to ensure rUTI will not return.

Lifestyle prevention strategies aim to reduce the frequency of infections:

- Ensure high-fluid intake
- Post-coital voiding, wiping front to back, limit perineal detergent hygiene use
- Cautious use of lubricants or spermicides.

Antibiotic Prophylaxis

Continuous low-dose antibiotic prophylaxis has consistently been shown to be superior than placebo or no treatment in the prevention of rUTI.

The therapy works by eliminating introital reservoirs of pathogenic bacteria.

Prescribed in the form of one tablet every night, common options include oral trimethoprim 100mg, cefalexin 125–250mg (PO), nitrofurantoin 50–100mg (PO).

Selected antibiotic will depend on local resistance patterns.

Antimicrobial prophylaxis can also be used as a post-coital preventive strategy.

Breakthrough infections should be treated with a different antibiotic (based on sensitivities) and prophylaxis resumed after acute treatment.

There is no consensus about the optimal duration of continuous antibiotic; however, 3–6 months is standard (NICE recommends reviewing after 6 months duration).

Screening for asymptomatic bacteriuria and providing antibiotic prophylaxis is not recommended in diabetics, neurogenic LUTS patients (e.g. MS) or those with indwelling catheters.

Topical Oestrogen

EAU 2024 recommends vaginal oestrogen replacement in post-menopausal women to prevent rUTI.

NICE recommends consider lowest effective dose of vaginal oestrogen for post-menopausal women with rUTI, if conservative management insufficient, via shared decision-making process. [31]

NICE and EAU both do not support use of oral oestrogen for rUTI prevention.

The long-term endometrial safety remains uncertain; any vaginal bleeding should be promptly reported.

Prescribed regime as per BNF includes oestrogen cream daily for 2/52, then twice weekly for 2/12, then discontinue for 4 weeks and reassess clinical need.

D-mannose

D-mannose is a plant extract which prevents bacterial adhesion to the bladder-wall cell surface thus contributing to barrier function; it can be bought over the counter.

Prophylaxis with 2g daily dose for ≤ 6 months can be offered to patients for rUTI prevention.

Patients should be counselled that evidence supporting its use is weak (NICE and EAU 2024).

Cranberry Supplementation

Cranberries contain proanthocyanidins which can inhibit adherence of P-pili E.coli to uroepithelial cell receptors. [32]

Patients should be counselled that evidence supporting its use is weak (NICE and EAU 2024).

Probiotics

Probiotics (lactobacillus) work via various different mechanisms, including inhibiting growth of their competitors, anti-adhesion properties and immune modulation.

Patients should be counselled that evidence supporting their use is weak (NICE and EAU 2024).

Self-treatment

In patients with good compliance, self-treatment with a short antibiotic regimen is an option.

Patients encouraged to take MSU sample prior to taking antibiotics, and proceed to same course and agent as per a standard acute UTI.

Methenamine Hippurate

Methenamine hippurate is absorbed in the gastro-intestinal tract and excreted by the kidneys to form methenamine and hippuric acid.

Methenamine is hydrolysed to bacteriostatic agents; hippuric acid ensures urinary pH remains acidic.

Can be prescribed as 1g Hiprex twice daily.

EAU 2024 recommends usage for rUTI prevention provided no structural abnormalities in urinary tract.

KEY PAPER | ALTAR Trial (2021) [33]

- Multi-centre, randomised, UK-based trial for women ≥ 18 years with rUTI needing prevention.
- 240 patients randomised 1:1 to receive (antibiotic prophylaxis) vs. (methenamine Hippurate).
- Primary outcome was incidence of symptomatic UTI requiring antibiotics.
- Trial demonstrated non-inferiority of methenamine with respect to antibiotic prophylaxis.

EPIDIDYMO-ORCHITIS

Acute inflammation of the epididymis, often involving the testis, usually due to bacterial infection.

Epididymitis can be acute, chronic or recurrent.

PATHOGENESIS

Infection ascends from the urethra or bladder.

In sexually active men aged < 35 years, common pathogens are N.gonorrhoeae and C.trachomatis, where a urethritis ascends to infect the epididymis.

In older men and children, the most common pathogen is E.coli.

In older men the most likely underlying cause is an ascending UTI as a result of BOO – recurrent episodes of epididymo-orchitis should prompt a full LUTS assessment.

m.TB is a rarer cause of epididymitis where the epididymis feels like a beaded cord.

Non-infective epididymitis may arise from amiodarone, which accumulates in the epididymis causing inflammation – this will resolve on interruption of the drug.

DIAGNOSTIC EVALUATION

Patient *history* should enquire regarding:

- Time and onset of scrotal pain/swelling
- Previous episodes and treatment/past urological history
- Sexual risk history and previous STI.

Patient *examination* (main differential diagnosis is testicular torsion) should evaluate for:

- Spermatic cord thickening and tenderness, rather than testicular findings
- Scrotal erythema or swelling
- Urethral discharge
- *Prehn's sign* (positive if hemi-scrotal elevation relieves symptoms, suggests epididymitis).

Testicular torsion features acute pain and swelling localised to the testis, whereas epididymitis is mainly preceded by infective symptoms with pain and swelling confined to epididymis.

If clinical diagnostic doubt remains, surgical exploration is mandatory.

Urinalysis with MSU culture and sensitivities should be performed.

If there is no urethral discharge for collection, then first voided urine for PCR to detect chlamydia.

US scrotum indicated, may show increased Doppler flow around epididymis (and testis).

MANAGEMENT

Patient should be resuscitated in systematic Airway-to-Exposure manner, ensuring that the Sepsis-6 bundle has been completed.

Antibiotic prescription directed by local guidelines and likely pathogen (based on patient age).

Any suspicion/confirmation of STI should prompt sexual health discussion with the patient and contact tracing as required.

Prescribe analgesia and anti-inflammatories +/- PPI cover.

Doxycycline covers chlamydial infection (azithromycin 1g stat if allergic as alternative), whilst ciprofloxacin covers gonococcal infection.

Persisting/worsening symptoms should prompt sonographic assessment for scrotal abscess, which may require urgent incision and drainage.

Mumps Orchitis

Mumps orchitis occurs in 30% of infected post-pubertal males, starting 5–7 days after onset of parotitis and can result in testicular atrophy.

10% of cases are bilateral and can cause infertility.

Management is supportive including scrotal support, ice packs, NSAIDs.

Mumps is a notifiable disease within the UK.

FOURNIER'S GANGRENE

Fournier's gangrene is a type-1 necrotising fasciitis of the external genitalia and perineum.

Most commonly occurs in men.

Overall mortality 20% (higher in diabetics, alcoholics and immuno-compromised).

PATHOPHYSIOLOGY

Infection most commonly arises from the skin, urethra or anorectal regions.

Synergistic microbial action such that multiple aerobic/anaerobic organisms are present, most commonly E.coli, often facultative organisms (e.g. Klebsiella, Enterococci, Clostridia).

Risk factors include:

- Recent instrumentation/catheterisation/penoscrotal surgery
- Diabetes
- LTC in situ
- Reduced mobility, elderly and infirm, immuno-compromised.

Infection spread is through local fascia, producing tissue necrosis and pus by anaerobes.

Degree of internal necrosis is usually greater than suggested by external signs.

DIAGNOSTIC EVALUATION

Patient *history* must enquire regarding:

- Time of onset and relative distribution of perineal changes
- Risk factors including long-term catheter, recent urological surgery, diabetes, infirmity
- Patient continence.

Patient *examination* should evaluate for:

- Fever and vital parameters assessment
- Focused urological: perineal swelling, oedema, erythema, tenderness, palpable crepitus
- Signs of necrosis or gangrene.

Cultures should be taken from relevant sources (urine, blood, groin pus).

Arterial blood gases and FBC, UE and CRP should be obtained.

Fournier's gangrene is a clinical diagnosis – imaging is not routinely required.

Fournier's Gangrene Severity Index

Mortality from Fournier's gangrene can be assessed via the Fournier's Gangrene Severity Index (Laor scoring system). [34]

This is a scoring system assigning points based on various parameters, including:

- Temperature, heart rate, respiratory rate
- Serum sodium/potassium/creatinine/bicarbonate
- Leucocyte count
- Haematocrit.

MANAGEMENT

The patient should be resuscitated in a systematic manner as per Airway-to-Exposure protocol, ensuring the Sepsis-6 bundle has been completed.

Adopt multi-disciplinary approach to liaise with critical care, microbiology and anaesthetics.

Broad-spectrum antibiotics should be given immediately with early involvement of microbiologist (often triple: co-amoxiclav, metronidazole and gentamicin).

Glycaemic control should be closely monitored and optimised.

Patient should be transferred to theatre without delay and consented for:

- Debridement of all necrotic tissue until healthy margins reached
- Potential need for urinary diversion in form of SPC
- Potential faecal diversion in form of colostomy
- Wound should be left open (with scheduled re-look within 24 hours)
- Blood transfusion, DVT/PE, death.

Testes are usually spared as their blood supply is independent and distinct.

Long-term healing is good; however, may require involvement of plastic surgery team.

EAU 2024 does not recommend use of hyperbaric oxygen in treating Fournier's gangrene.

PROSTATITIS

EPIDEMIOLOGY

Prostatitis is relatively common; however, < 10% cases have proven bacterial infection.

E.coli is the most common pathogen featuring in acute bacterial prostatitis, in CBP the spectrum is wider, in HIV/immunosuppression organisms such as m.TB or candida may feature.

CBP is defined where patient symptoms persist > 3 months.

Risk factors are those predisposing to genito-urinary tract and prostatic bacterial colonisation:

- UTI/epididymitis
- Trans-urethral surgery/indwelling catheters
- Prostatic stones
- Immunosuppression.

DIAGNOSTIC EVALUATION

Patient *history* should enquire regarding:

- Fevers, chills, rigors, general malaise (acute presentation)
- rUTI, ejaculatory problems, chronic pain (chronic presentation)
- Pain is poorly localised but commonly around the saddle area
- LUTS
- Previous prostatitis/chronicity of symptoms/known urological history.

Patient *examination* should evaluate for:

- Lower abdominal tenderness or palpable bladder
- DRE for tender and/or swollen prostate (fluctuant feeling prostate suggests abscess).

Haematospermia in men in endemic TB regions should be investigated for urinary TB (ejaculate analysis, however, is not recommended for microbial investigations).

Prostatic massage in the acute presentation not recommended (risk of bacteraemia and/or sepsis).

Collect blood tests for FBC, UE, CRP and blood cultures if patient is febrile or septic.

Perform urinalysis (check for nitrites and leucocytes) and send MSU culture.

Consider sending urine to test for gonorrhoea and chlamydia.

Imaging

Consider US KUB to evaluate for urinary retention, PVR and hydronephrosis.

To evaluate for prostatic abscess, options include CT abdomen/pelvis or TRUS.

Meares and Stamey Test

Meares and Stamey 4-glass test is standard method of assessing presence of bacteria in the lower urinary tract in men presenting with symptoms of chronic prostatitis.

Rarely used in routine clinical practice due to time and difficulty performing it.

The test is performed as follows (full bladder and no ejaculations > 3 days): [28]

- (VB1) 10mL of first-voided urine (positive culture indicates urethritis/ prostatitis), then
- (VB2) 100mL of voided urine from bladder (positive culture indicates cystitis), then
- (EPS) massage prostate for 60 seconds, collect secretions from urethra (positive culture indicates prostatitis), then
- (VB3) 10mL of voided urine after massage (positive culture indicates prostatitis).

Where cultures are negative, increased numbers of leucocytes per high-powered field (> 10) on microscopy favours a diagnosis of CPPS.

EAU 2024 recommends using classification by NIDDK in which bacterial prostatitis is distinguished from CPPS (Table 9).

Alpha-blockers may have therapeutic value in patients with category III (not as monotherapy).

Category IV requires no further investigations or treatment.

Table 9 – Classification of prostatitis and CPPS as per NIDDK [29]

Type	Name and Description
I	Acute bacterial prostatitis
II	Chronic bacterial prostatitis
III	Chronic abacterial prostatitis – CPPS
IIIA	Inflammatory CPPS (WBCs in EPS / post-prostatic massage urine / semen)
IIIB	Non-inflammatory CPPS (no white cells seen)
IV	Asymptomatic inflammatory prostatitis (histological prostatitis)

MANAGEMENT

Acute Prostatitis

In the acutely ill patient, resuscitate in systematic Airway-to-Exposure manner, completing the Sepsis-6 bundle and liaise with critical care and microbiology.

Antibiotic choice will be guided by local protocols, however:

- EAU 2024 recommends fluoroquinolones first-line agents
- Antibiotic duration is extended course (minimum 14 days).

Prostatic abscess can be managed conservatively or drained, which can be done percutaneously, TRUS guided or via trans-urethral approach in theatre.

Chronic Prostatitis

EAU 2024 recommends fluoroquinolone (e.g. ciprofloxacin, levofloxacin) as first-line treatment agent for an extended duration (4–6 weeks).

Consider prescribing α-blocker to promote smooth muscle relaxation.

The lower urinary tract should be investigated from a functional point of view (uroflowmetry, PVR) and any relevant findings should be addressed (e.g. BOO, chronic retention).

KIDNEY INFECTIONS

DEFINITIONS

Pyelonephritis is inflammation of the kidney and renal pelvis.

Uncomplicated pyelonephritis is defined as pyelonephritis limited to non-pregnant, pre-menopausal women with no known functional or anatomical urological abnormalities

Pyonephrosis – infected hydronephrosis as pus accumulates within the renal pelvis/calyces.

Peri-nephric abscess develops as a consequence of extension of infection outside of the kidney parenchyma during acute pyelonephritis.

Emphysematous pyelonephritis – acute necrotising pyelonephritis by gas-forming organisms.

Emphysematous pyelitis describes presence of gas limited to renal excretory system.

ACUTE PYELONEPHRITIS

EPIDEMIOLOGY

1–2 per 1,000 women are affected each year (0.5 per 1,000 males).

More common in pregnant (1–4%) vs. non-pregnant women, and will occur in ≤ 25% of pregnant women who have untreated bacteriuria. [35]

Most cases of acute pyelonephritis start off as lower UTI.

Most commonly due to bacterial infection of E.coli (80%) due to P-pili virulence factors.

Risk factors include diabetes, pregnancy, sexual activity, recent urinary tract instrumentation, VUR, urinary tract obstruction and indwelling catheters.

PATHOGENESIS

80% due to E.coli, other organisms include Enterococci, Klebsiella, Proteus and Pseudomonas.

Any process interfering with ureteric peristalsis (i.e. obstruction) may assist in retrograde bacterial ascent from bladder to kidney.

Initially there is patchy infiltration of neutrophils and bacteria in the parenchyma; later changes include formation of inflammatory bands extending from renal papilla to cortex.

DIAGNOSTIC EVALUATION

Patient *history* should enquire regarding:

- Preceding LUTS/cystitis/recent use of antibiotics
- Loin pain and/or VH (may suggest urolithiasis)
- Fever/chills/rigors (swinging fever may suggest pyonephrosis)
- Previous pyelonephritis episodes/past urological history/known stone former
- Underlying conditions that may compromise patient immunity.

Patient *examination* with chaperone should assess for:

- Abdominal examination for suprapubic/renal angle tenderness
- Fever, vital parameters, signs of sepsis.

Perform urinalysis to assess for infection and NVH and send MSU for culture.

Collect blood tests to include FBC, UE, CRP and blood cultures if febrile or sepsis is suspected.

Imaging

US KUB may be preferred in young females of child-bearing age to evaluate for urolithiasis, urinary obstruction, hydronephrosis or abscess/collection.

Alternatively CT KUB can be requested first line if high index of suspicion of underlying stone pathology or the patient is acutely unwell.

Persisting/swinging fever should prompt repeat imaging to evaluate for renal abscess.

DMSA is the most reliable test for diagnosing pyelonephritis; however, rarely used first line in UK.

MANAGEMENT

Resuscitate patient in systematic manner via Airway-to-Exposure approach, ensuring the Sepsis-6 bundle has been completed.

IV antibiotics are recommended for patients requiring hospitalisation.

Antibiotic choice should be broad-spectrum and in line with local guidelines; IV duration may be short until patient clinically improves after which oral step-down should be considered.

Any abscess/pyonephrosis should be urgently drained percutaneously by IR.

Routine post-treatment urinalysis or cultures are not required in asymptomatic patients, except in pregnant women, as eradication of bacteriuria should be achieved.

PERINEPHRIC ABSCESS

Perinephric abscesses develop as a consequence of extension of infection outside the parenchyma of the kidney during acute pyelonephritis and accumulates within Gerota's fascia.

A perinephric abscess may therefore arise from:

- Rupture of cortical abscess
- Failure to achieve drainage of pyonephrosis
- Haematogenous spread of infection from distant site.

Risk factors include diabetes, immuno-compromised status and obstructing ureteric calculi.

Causative organisms include S.aureus (Gram positive), E.coli, Proteus (Gram negative).

DIAGNOSTIC EVALUATION

Patient *history* as per acute pyelonephritis; in addition, should evaluate for:

- Symptom duration > 5 days (compared to < 5 days seen in acute pyelonephritis)
- Pyelonephritis symptoms not resolving despite ≥ 4 days of IV antibiotics, which should raise the suspicion of pus accumulation in or around the kidney.

Patient *examination* as per acute pyelonephritis; in addition, should evaluate for:

- Flank mass with overlying skin erythema
- Hip extension may trigger pain (psoas spasm).

MANAGEMENT

Resuscitate patient in systematic manner via Airway-to-Exposure approach, ensuring the Sepsis-6 bundle has been completed.

Request CTU to evaluate size and location of abscess.

The key intervention is the urgent percutaneous IR-guided drainage of pus from the kidney; open drainage is rarely required.

Nephrectomy may be required for extensive involvement or non-functioning kidney.

EMPHYSEMATOUS PYELONEPHRITIS

Rare form of acute necrotising pyelonephritis caused by gas-forming organisms, with radiographic evidence of gas within or around the kidney. [36]

Most cases are associated with underlying poorly controlled diabetes (> 90% of cases).

Other associated conditions may be urinary tract obstruction, stones, impaired immunity.

High levels of glucose in poorly controlled diabetics provide an ideal environment for fermentation by enterobacteria, producing CO_2.

There is an associated overwhelming inflammatory response, and due to diabetic microangiopathy the end products are not transported away. [28]

EPN is most commonly caused by E.coli and klebsiella.

DIAGNOSTIC EVALUATION

Presents as per acute pyelonephritis (high fever, flank pain, malaise) but likely will be critically ill, or deteriorate despite resuscitation and antibiotic therapy.

Urgent CT with contrast should be requested.

Grading

EPN can be graded radiologically:

- *Type 1*, destruction > 1/3 of parenchyma with either absence of fluid collection or presence of gas radiating from medulla to cortex (mortality ≤ 60%)

- *Type 2*, destruction < 1/3 of parenchyma, confined intra-renal gas pattern, presence of renal/perirenal gas within collecting system, renal collections may be present (mortality ≤ 20%).

Alternatively *Huang and Tseng* EPN classification can be used:

1. Gas in collecting system only

2. Parenchymal gas only

3. (A) extension of gas into perinephric space (B) extension of gas into pararenal space

4. EPN in solitary kidney or bilateral disease.

MANAGEMENT

Resuscitate patient in systematic manner via Airway-to-Exposure approach, ensuring the Sepsis-6 bundle has been completed; liaise early with critical care team.

Patients are often critically ill at presentation and will require transfer to HDU/ITU for support.

Mainstay of management is supportive, antibiotics, fluids and percutaneous IR-guided drainage.

If patient fails to improve despite resuscitation, consider repeat CT in view of draining other pockets of infection and rediscussing with microbiologist in view of adjusting antibiotic therapy.

Further deterioration may necessitate consideration of emergency nephrectomy.

XANTHOGRANULOMATOUS PYELONEPHRITIS

XGP is a severe renal infection resulting in diffuse parenchymal destruction and non-functioning kidney, usually associated with underlying stone disease. [37]

Severe form of chronic pyelonephritis which tends to present sub-acutely, rather than acutely unwell.

Proteus is the most common causative organism (E.coli less common).

Gas formation is not a feature.

Occurs more often in women.

Broad management principles similar to EPN – however, patient less likely to be critically ill, nephrectomy advisable due to symptom chronicity and radiological challenge of excluding RCC.

PATHOLOGY

Microscopically appears as diffuse infiltration of inflammatory cells (e.g. lymphocytes, giant cells) with the characteristic finding of xanthoma cells (lipid-laden macrophages or foam cells).

Macroscopically appears as an enlarged kidney with yellow nodules of pus and areas of necrosis.

Radiologically may be challenging to distinguish from RCC (i.e. histology required).

DIAGNOSTIC EVALUATION

Patient may present with flank pain, fever, VH and tender flank mass.

Complications include fistulae formation (nephrocolonic, nephrocutaneous), psoas abscess.

Collect blood tests for FBC, UE, CRP, INR (likely to require percutaneous drainage).

Blood and MSU cultures should be collected.

Imaging

US will reveal enlarged kidney with echogenic material.

CT is investigation of choice; may feature cortical thinning, perinephric fat inflammation, hydronephrosis or nephrolithiasis (*bear paw abnormality*). [38]

DMSA likely to reveal poorly or non-functioning kidney.

CHRONIC PELVIC PAIN

CPPS is chronic or persistent pain perceived in structures related to the pelvis in men and women, where there is no proven local pathology/infection to account for symptom.

CPPS often associated with negative cognitive, behavioural, sexual and emotional consequences.

Aetiology of CPPS is poorly understood and likely multifactorial, including low-grade infection, chemical irritation, altered immunity and neuromuscular disturbances.

If the pain is localised to single organ, this can be defined as primary (organ) pain syndrome (e.g. primary prostate pain syndrome, primary epididymal pain syndrome).

DIAGNOSTIC EVALUATION

Patient *history* should enquire regarding:

- Duration of symptoms, impact on QOL, most bothersome symptoms
- Previous medical or surgical treatments for condition (or pelvic conditions)
- Urinary/bowel/sexual symptoms
- Psychological history and wellbeing.

Formal evaluation with Chronic Prostatitis Symptom Index questionnaire is encouraged.

Patient *examination* with chaperone should evaluate:

- Abdomen for anatomical abnormality (palpable kidney/bladder)
- DRE for prostate pain/tenderness
- External genitalia for scrotal pain/tenderness.

Perform urinalysis, collect MSU for culture.

Further investigations are guided by organ-specific symptoms (e.g. uroflowmetry, UDS, cystoscopy, semen culture, STI screen).

Potassium chloride sensitivity test (*Parson's test*) consists of instilling potassium chloride into bladder via catheter, which may yield pain/cystitis symptoms (gauges permeability of GAG layer).

This test alone has a poor sensitivity and specificity. [39]

UPOINTS

Urology, Psychology, Organ specific, Infection, Neurological, Tender muscle, Sexological [29]

UPOINTS phenotype classification can classify patients with an established diagnosis of CPPS into a clinically relevant phenotype that can guide therapy.

UPOINTS is not designed to diagnose these conditions.

PROSTATE PAIN SYNDROME

PPS is persistent or recurrent pain which is convincingly reproduced by prostatic palpation.

The term chronic prostatitis is often used interchangeably but is no longer preferred.

PPS assessment should employ Meares and Stamey 4-glass test (see "Prostatitis" section).

The diagnosis of PPS on the 4-glass test is established if:

- VB1 (first-voided urine) and VB2 (bladder urine) specimens are sterile
- EPS and VB3 (post-massage urine) < 10,000 CFU bacteria and insignificant leucocytes.

Presence of organisms/leucocytes in EPS or VB3 specimens indicate possible chronic prostatitis.

An alternative method is *Nickel's pre- and post-massage test*, involving urine microscopy of pre- and post-massage samples (PPS possible if post-massage sample negative).

The classification of prostatitis is discussed in the prostatitis section.

TREATMENT

Antibiotics, NSAIDs and α-blockers are cornerstone of management.

Quinolones (e.g. ciprofloxacin) or tetracyclines (e.g. doxycycline) are preferred in PPS due to good penetration and bioavailability within prostate, treatment duration ≤ 6 weeks.

NSAIDs can be offered in addition to antibiotics (consider PPI cover alongside).

α-blockers can be offered if antibiotic therapy is unsuccessful.

Alternatives to NSAIDs include tricyclic antidepressants, diazepam or baclofen.

BLADDER PAIN SYNDROME

BPS is the presence of persistent or recurrent pain perceived in the urinary bladder region > 6 months, accompanied by ≥ 1 other urinary symptom.

There is no proven infection or other obvious pathology.

The term interstitial cystitis is no longer recommended for use.

BPS is a diagnosis of exclusion.

Anti-proliferative factor is produced by bladder urothelium, potential mediator of BPS by increasing transmembrane permeability and decreasing heparin-binding epidermal growth factor. [40]

Classification

Classification of BPS is based on cystoscopy and hydrodistension (+/- bladder biopsy).

Glomerulations are pin-point red marks on bladder wall (petechial haemorrhages).

Hunner's ulcers are lesions described as circumscribed red areas with small vessels radiating toward central scar with attached fibrin deposit and central fragility.

LASER fulguration of Hunner's ulcers can provide symptomatic relief.

Positive biopsy implies inflammatory and/or granulation tissue and/or detrusor mastocytosis.

MANAGEMENT

A holistic approach to the BPS patient is advised, working alongside a pain specialist, psychosocial counselling and support group.

Bladder instillations can be used to restore the GAG layer.

URETHRITIS

Urethral inflammation usually presents with LUTS; must be distinguished from other infections.

From therapeutic and clinical point of view, urethritis should be categorised as: [29]

- Gonorrhoeal urethritis
- Non-gonococcal urethritis.

Other pathogens include C.trachomatis, Mycoplasma genitalium, T.vaginalis.

Pathogens remain extracellularly on the epithelial layer or penetrate into the epithelium and cause pyogenic infection.

Chlamydia and gonorrhoea can spread further across urogenital tract to affect epididymis in men and endometrium and fallopian tubes in women.

DIAGNOSTIC EVALUATION

Patient *history* should enquire regarding:

- Dysuria, urinary symptoms, pain in penile shaft or meatus
- Urethral discharge
- Sexual history and previous STI.

Patient *examination* with chaperone should evaluate for:

- External genitalia for tenderness, rash, lesions or discharge
- Fever and vital parameters.

Collect MSU for culture, 20mL of first-voided urine to test for chlamydia and gonorrhoea (NAAT).

A Gram stain of urethral discharge or urethral smear showing ≥ 5 leucocytes/HPF and gonococci located intracellularly indicates gonococcal urethritis.

Consider consenting patient for HIV and venereal disease testing.

MANAGEMENT

Manage patient with active involvement from microbiology and genito-urinary medicine teams.

Gonorrhoeal urethritis can be treated with ceftriaxone 1g IM stat + azithromycin 1g PO stat.

Non-gonococcal urethritis without identified pathogen can be treated with doxycycline 100mg PO BD for 7 days or azithromycin.

If GU treated with single-dose therapy but patient does not improve clinically or symptoms recur within days, consider additional treatment for C.trachomatis (most common cause).

Contact tracing should be undertaken.

URINARY TRACT INFECTIONS IN PREGNANCY

EPIDEMIOLOGY

5% of pregnant women have asymptomatic bacteriuria (same as background population of young women); however, ≤ 25% of these will progress to develop pyelonephritis.

With correct antibiotic treatment the risk of pyelonephritis reduces to ≤ 5%.

EAU 2024 – pregnant women should have asymptomatic bacteriuria treated. [29]

Short course of antibiotics is recommended rather than CAP.

MANAGEMENT

Antibiotic choice must bear in mind pregnancy status, allergies and antimicrobial sensitivities.

Penicillins and cephalosporins are considered safe antibiotics for use during pregnancy.

Antibiotics to avoid during pregnancy include:

- First trimester: trimethoprim (folate deficiency)
- Second and third trimester: aminoglycosides
- All trimesters: quinolones, tetracyclines.

Once antibiotic course is completed, a repeat MSU must be performed to confirm eradication of bacteria, in contrast to uncomplicated UTI scenario where this is not necessary.

For rUTI in pregnancy – consider low dose (125–250mg) cephalexin daily as CAP.

URINARY SCHISTOSOMIASIS

Urinary schistosomiasis is also called bilharzia.

Most commonly found in Africa, Asia and South America.

PATHOPHYSIOLOGY

Schistosomiasis is caused by the parasitic trematode/flatworm *Schistosoma haematobium* (other organisms include S.mansoni and S.japonicum).

Infection is acquired by exposure to contaminated water.

The parasites (cercariae) penetrate the skin of host, shed their tails and migrate to the liver to mature.

Adult worms then travel to veins of vesical plexus and lay fertilised eggs, which can:

- Penetrate bladder and enter urine
- Remain trapped in tissues and become calcified eosinophilic granuloma (T-cell response).

The disease has two main stages:

- *Active*, when adult worms are laying eggs (eggs are immunogenic and cause symptoms)
- *Inactive*, adults have died and there is a reaction to remaining eggs.

Eggs are then shed to be up taken in fresh water by the intermediate host snail.

The intermediate host snail is specific:

- Bulinus for *S.haematobium*
- Biomphalaria for *S.mansoni*.

You may be asked in the FRCS (Urol) viva to draw the life cycle of schistosomiasis (Figure 4).

Ureteric involvement complicates ≤ 25% of cases of bladder schistosomiasis, is usually bilateral and most commonly affects the distal ureter.

> **VIVA**   You may be asked in the FRCS (Urol) viva to draw the life cycle of schistosomiasis (Figure 4) – you must know how to reproduce this scheme efficiently and confidently.

Figure 4 – Life cycle of schistosomiasis

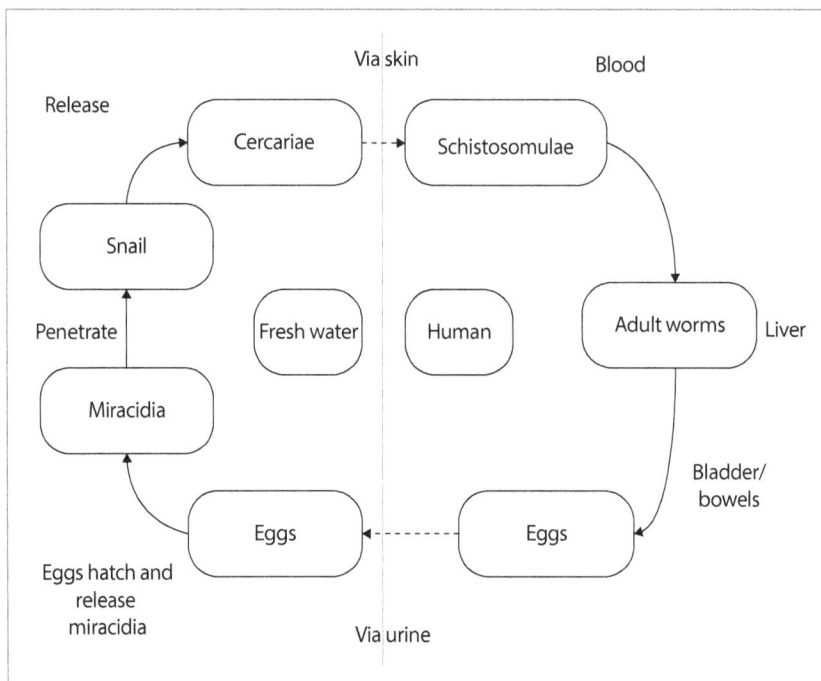

DIAGNOSTIC EVALUATION

The first symptom may be dermatitis at the site of entry of parasite (*swimmer's itch*).

Followed by *Katayama fever*, a generalised immune reaction associated with onset of egg-laying to include fever, malaise, lymphadenopathy, hepatosplenomegaly (3–12 weeks).

Urinary schistosomiasis may lead to delayed VH (e.g. after 12 weeks) and terminal dysuria.

Collect bloods for FBC (may reveal raised eosinophil count), UE, CRP and cultures.

Request imaging – US KUB may reveal hydronephrosis and/or thickened bladder wall, CTU may show a calcified, contracted bladder.

Urine collection is recommended between noon and 3pm to maximise chance of detecting eggs (distinguished by terminal spine).

Eggs may also be found in faeces.

Consider flexible cystoscopy (may reveal sandy patches of eggs on trigone) or bladder/rectal biopsy to confirm presence of eggs.

MANAGEMENT

Resuscitate patient in systematic manner via Airway-to-Exposure approach, ensuring the Sepsis-6 bundle has been completed; liaise with infectious diseases team.

Praziquantel 40mg/kg as a single or divided dose (cure rate 85–100%) (if fails, repeat dose).

Steroids can be used to treat Katayama fever stage.

Long-term sequalae may include:

- Fibrosis/eggshell calcification of the bladder which will lead to reduced compliance
- Hydronephrosis or upper-tract compromise
- Increased risk of SCCa of the bladder.

Therefore consider long-term follow-up to include:

- Monitoring of renal function via blood tests for UE
- Lifelong annual flexible cystoscopy surveillance of bladder
- Monitoring of upper tract via US KUB.

URINARY TUBERCULOSIS

EPIDEMIOLOGY

TB is predominantly seen in Asian populations.

Higher incidence in males compared to females. [41]

The kidney is the most common site of extra-pulmonary TB.

In the genital tract, primary site of involvement is epididymis (males) and fallopian tubes (females).

PATHOGENESIS

TB of the genito-urinary tract is caused by Mycobacterium tuberculosis.

M.bovis, M.africanum and M.microti can also cause TB.

Usually acquired by inhalation of infected droplets causing bacilli deposition in lungs (*primary TB*).

In primary TB, a granulomatous lesion forms in the mid-/upper zone of the lung; a central area of caseation necrosis surrounded by Langhans and epithelioid cells.

In immuno-competent individuals this process is self-limiting and sub-clinical.

Acute systemic dissemination of TB can, however, result in symptomatic *miliary TB*.

Post-primary TB is latent reactivation of infection which occurs at a time of host immuno-compromise, which will lead to clinical manifestations (25% of worldwide deaths in HIV patients is due to TB).

Lifetime risk of TB reactivation is 10%.

The spread of TB infection from lungs to urinary system is haematogenous (to the kidney), from where subsequently by direct extension it can pass to ureters and bladder.

The pathognomic lesion of TB is the caseating granuloma.

This comprises Langhans giant cells surrounded by lymphocytes and fibroblasts, and the healing of these lesions causes fibrosis and calcification.

DIAGNOSTIC EVALUATION

Patient *history* should specifically enquire regarding:

- Risk factors for TB – ethnic background, foreign travel, crowded accommodation
- Lethargy, weight loss, night sweats, fevers, haemoptysis
- rUTI not responding to treatment
- Comorbidities such as HIV, steroid use and diabetes mellitus.

Patient *examination* with chaperone should include:

- Chest and abdominal examination
- Palpable lymphadenopathy
- Genital examination.

Collect MSU (may reveal sterile pyuria), consider cytology to exclude other causes (e.g. CIS).

CXR may show granulomas, sputum culture should be sent.

Tuberculin Skin Test

Involves an intra-dermal injection of protein derivative of m.TB.

A positive result suggests exposure to TB (not necessarily active infection); however, a negative result excludes the diagnosis of TB.

Urine TB Culture

m.TB is not suitable for standard Gram-stain testing due to high lipid content of the cell wall.

m.TB is present intermittently in the urine, collect ≥ 3 early morning samples on consecutive days for analysis to increase likelihood of positive yield.

The smear of the urine is tested using *Ziehl–Neelsen* stain looking for acid-fast bacilli which will stain pink (non-acid fast bacilli stain purple).

The specimen is also cultured using the *Lowenstein–Jensen* culture medium; however, it is slow growing and may take ≤ 8 weeks to yield a result.

Imaging

CTU is the radiological investigation of choice, as it allows visualisation of anatomy, strictures, calcification and parenchymal destruction.

CXR should also be requested looking for granulomatous lesions.

Cystoscopy

Patients may have haematuria or voiding LUTS which warrant a diagnostic cystoscopy anyway.

TB of bladder may appear as areas of bullous oedema, ulceration and haemorrhage, and these can be biopsied and cauterised.

EFFECTS ON GENITO-URINARY TRACT

The first spread from the lungs is via the bloodstream to the kidneys, where it then may spread by direct extension to the rest of the urinary tract.

Kidney

Granuloma formation in renal cortex and caseous necrosis of renal papillae, leading to bacilli release into the urine.

Healing fibrosis and calcification leads to shrunken irregular kidney or *auto-nephrectomy*.

Poorly compliant bladder may jeopardise upper-tract function.

Ureters

Ureteric strictures in TB are common, and may be multiple or complex.

VUR is also common due to the distortion of the ureteric orifices.

Bladder

Spread to the bladder is usually via direct extension from the kidney; however, it can be acquired iatrogenically via intra-vesical BCG treatment.

Bladder wall becomes oedematous, red, inflamed (yellow lesions with red halo) and the characteristic fibrosis healing leads to small contracted, poorly compliant bladder.

Prostate/Seminal Vesicles

Haematogenous spread creates hard irregular calcifications.

Epididymis

Spread can be haematogenous or from kidney, the affected epididymis may feel like a beaded cord on examination, and this is usually unilateral.

Abscesses and infertility are potential further complications.

MANAGEMENT

The patient is best managed in a multi-disciplinary team setting with input from urology, microbiology, respiratory and infectious diseases teams.

Mainstay of management is multi-drug anti-TB regimens.

Typical combination is RIPE (rifampicin, isoniazid, pyrazinamide, ethambutol) for 2 months, and further 4 months of rifampicin and isoniazid.

Steroids not routinely indicated unless for ureteric stricture not responding to anti-TB medication.

Multi-drug-resistant TB strains are becoming increasingly prevalent

REFERENCES

1. Reynard J, Brewster S, Biers S (2009). *Oxford Handbook of Urology*, second edition, Oxford University Press, Oxford.
2. Hyun JS (2018). Clinical significance of prostatic calculi: a review. *World Journal of Men's Health*, *36*(1), 15–21.
3. Ratkalkar VN, Kleinman JG (2011). Mechanisms of stone formation. *Clinical Reviews in Bone and Mineral Metabolism*, *9*(3–4), 187–197.
4. Evan AP, Lingeman JE, Coe FL (2003). Randall's plaque of patients with nephrolithiasis begins in basement membranes of thin loops of Henle. *Journal of Clinical Investigation*, *111*(5), 607–616.
5. Hueppelshaeuser R, von Unruh GE, Habbig S (2012). Enteric hyperoxaluria, recurrent urolithiasis, and systemic oxalosis in patients with Crohn's disease. *Pediatric Nephrology*, *27*(7), 1,103–1,109.
6. NICE Guidelines (2019). Renal and ureteric stones: assessment and management. Available at: https://www.nice.org.uk/guidance/ng118/resources/renal-and-ureteric-stones-assessment-and-management-pdf-66141605137093 [last accessed 8 August 2024].
7. Johnston T, Rochester M, Wiseman O (2018). Urinary Tract Stones. In: *Viva Practice for the FRCS (Urol) and Postgraduate Urology Examinations*, CRC Press, London.
8. Nakasato T, Morita J, Ogawa Y (2015). Evaluation of Hounsfield Units as a predictive factor for the outcome of extracorporeal shock wave lithotripsy and stone composition. *Urolithiasis*, *43*(1), 69–75.
9. Jung P, Brauers A, Nolte-Ernsting CA (2000). Magnetic resonance urography enhanced by gadolinium and diuretics: a comparison with conventional urography in diagnosing the cause of ureteric obstruction. *BJU International*, *86*(9), 960–965.
10. Skolarikos A, Jung H, Neisius A, et al. (2024). EAU Guidelines for Urolithiasis. Available at: https://d56bochluxqnz.cloudfront.net/documents/full-guideline/EAU-Guidelines-on-Urolithiasis-2024.pdf [last accessed 20 August 2024].
11. Holdgate A, Pollock T (2004). Systematic review of the relative efficacy of non-steroidal anti-inflammatory drugs and opioids in the treatment of acute renal colic. *BMJ*, *328*(7,453), 1,401.
12. Pearle MS, Pierce HL, Miller GL (1998). Optimal method of urgent decompression of the collecting system for obstruction and infection due to ureteral calculi. *Journal of Urology*, *160*(4), 1,260–1,264.
13. Glowacki LS, Beecroft ML, Cook RJ (1992). The natural history of asymptomatic urolithiasis. *Journal of Urology*, *147*(2), 319–321.

14. Dropkin BM, Moses R, Sharma D (2015). The natural history of nonobstructing asymptomatic renal stones managed with active surveillance. *Journal of Urology*, *193*(4), 1,265–1,269.

15. Pickard R, Starr K, MacLennan G (2015). Medical expulsive therapy in adults with ureteric colic: a multicentre, randomised, placebo-controlled trial. *Lancet*, *386*(9,991), 341–349.

16. Shah TT, Gao C, Peters M, et al. (2019). Factors associated with spontaneous stone passage in a contemporary cohort of patients presenting with acute ureteric colic: results from the Multi-centre cohort study evaluating the role of Inflammatory Markers in patients presenting with acute ureteric Colic (MIMIC). *BJU International*, *124*(3), 504–513.

17. Dasgupta R, Cameron S, Aucott L, et al. (2021). Shockwave Lithotripsy Versus Ureteroscopic Treatment as Therapeutic Interventions for Stones of the Ureter (TISU): a Multicentre Randomised Controlled Non-inferiority Trial. *European Urology*, *80*(1), 46–54.

18. Manikandan R, Gall Z, Gunendran T (2007). Do anatomic factors pose a significant risk in the formation of lower pole stones? *Urology*, *69*(4), 620–624.

19. Sumino Y, Mimata H, Tasaki Y (2002). Predictors of lower pole renal stone clearance after extracorporeal shock wave lithotripsy. *Journal of Urology*, *168*(4 Part 1), 1,344–1,347.

20. Albala DM, Assimos DG, Clayman RV (2001). Lower pole I: a prospective randomized trial of extracorporeal shock wave lithotripsy and percutaneous nephrostolithotomy for lower pole nephrolithiasis – initial results. *Journal of Urology*, *166*(6), 2,072–2,080.

21. Pearle MS, Lingeman JE, Leveillee R (2005). Prospective, randomized trial comparing shock wave lithotripsy and ureteroscopy for lower pole caliceal calculi 1 cm or less. *Journal of Urology*, *173*(6), 2,005–2,009.

22. Diri A, Diri B (2018). Management of staghorn renal stones. *Renal Failure*, *40*(1), 357–362.

23. Blandy JP, Singh M (1976). The case for a more aggressive approach to staghorn stones. *Journal of Urology*, *115*(5), 505–506.

24. Teichman JM, Long RD, Hulbert JC (1995). Long-term renal fate and prognosis after staghorn calculus management. *Journal of Urology*, *153*(5), 1,403–1,407.

25. Deutsch P, Subramonian K (2016). Conservative management of staghorn calculi: a single-centre experience. *BJU International*, 118(3), 444–450.

26. Hoppe B, von Unruh GE, Blank G (2005). Absorptive hyperoxaluria leads to an increased risk for urolithiasis or nephrocalcinosis in cystic fibrosis. *American Journal of Kidney Diseases*, *46*(3), 440–445.

27. Claes DJ, Jackson E (2012). Cystinuria: mechanisms and management. *Pediatric Nephrology, 27*(11), 2,031–2,038.

28. Mishra V, Kalsi JS (2018). Urinary tract infections. In: *Viva Practice for the FRCS (Urol) and Postgraduate Urology Examinations*, CRC Press, London.

29. Bonkat G, Bartoletti RR, Bruyere F, et al. (2024). EAU Guidelines on Urological Infections. Available at: https://d56bochluxqnz.cloudfront.net/documents/full-guideline/EAU-Guidelines-on-Urological-Infections-2024.pdf [last accessed 31 August 2024].

30. Sanchez GV, Fleming-Dutra KE, Roberts RM (2016). Core elements of outpatient antibiotic stewardship. *Morbidity and Mortality Weekly Report: Recommendations and Reports, 65*(6), 1–12.

31. NICE Guidelines (2018). Urinary tract infection (recurrent): antimicrobial prescribing. Available at: https://www.nice.org.uk/guidance/ng112/resources/urinary-tract-infection-recurrent-antimicrobial-prescribing-pdf-66141595059397 [last accessed 29 August 2024].

32. McMurdo ME, Bissett LY, Price RJ (2005). Does ingestion of cranberry juice reduce symptomatic urinary tract infections in older people in hospital? A double-blind, placebo-controlled trial. *Age and Ageing, 34*(3), 256–261.

33. Harding C, Mossop H, Homer T, et al. (2021). Alternative to prophylactic antibiotics for the treatment of recurrent urinary tract infections in women: multicentre, open label, randomised, non-inferiority trial. *BMJ, 376*.

34. Laor E, Palmer LS, Tolia BM (1995). Outcome prediction in patients with Fournier's gangrene. *Journal of Urology, 154*(1), 89–92.

35. Hill JB, Sheffield JS, McIntire DD (2005). Acute pyelonephritis in pregnancy. *Obstetrics & Gynecology, 105*(1), 18–23.

36. Huang JJ, Tseng CC (2000). Emphysematous pyelonephritis: clinicoradiological classification, management, prognosis, and pathogenesis. *Archives of Internal Medicine, 160*(6), 797–805.

37. Li L, Parwani AV (2011). Xanthogranulomatous pyelonephritis. *Archives of Pathology & Laboratory Medicine, 135*(5), 671–674.

38. Lee JH, Kim SS, Kim DS (2019). Xanthogranulomatous Pyelonephritis: "Bear's Paw Sign". *Journal of the Belgian Society of Radiology, 103*(1).

39. Sant GR (2002). Etiology, pathogenesis, and diagnosis of interstitial cystitis. *Reviews in Urology, 4*(S1), S9.

40. Kuo HC (2014). Potential urine and serum biomarkers for patients with bladder pain syndrome/interstitial cystitis. *International Journal of Urology, 21*, 34–41.

41. Figueiredo AA, Lucon AM, Junior RF (2008). Epidemiology of urogenital tuberculosis worldwide. *International Journal of Urology, 15*(9), 827–832.

CALCULI & URINARY TRACT INFECTIONS MCQS

1. Which of the following drugs is not recognised to be a potential cause of kidney stone formation?

    A) Sulphadiazine
    B) Atazanavir
    C) Indinavir
    D) Adalimumab
    E) Ceftriaxone

2. Which of the following stone compositions is given the mineral name of "whewellite"?

    A) Basic calcium phosphate
    B) Calcium oxalate monohydrate
    C) Calcium oxalate dihydrate
    D) Calcium hydroxyl phosphate
    E) Calcium carbonate

3. Which of the following is not a recognised inhibitor of stone formation?

    A) Magnesium
    B) Osteopontin
    C) Lipoprotein-A
    D) Prothrombin fragment 1
    E) Chondroitin sulfate

4. Which of the following stones is hexagonal in shape under microscopy?

    A) Cystine
    B) Uric acid
    C) Calcium oxalate monohydrate
    D) Calcium oxalate dihydrate
    E) Calcium phosphate

5. What is generally considered an optimal frequency of shockwaves during ESWL?

    A) 1–1.5Hz
    B) 2–2.5Hz
    C) 3–3.5Hz
    D) 4–4.5Hz
    E) 5–5.5Hz

6. *What is pure struvite made of?*

   A) Cystine ammonium calcium phosphate
   B) Oxalate ammonium calcium phosphate
   C) Oxalate ammonium phosphate
   D) Magnesium ammonium calcium phosphate
   E) Magnesium ammonium phosphate

7. *Which of the following antibiotics is considered safe in pregnancy?*

   A) Ceftriaxone
   B) Trimethoprim
   C) Nitrofurantoin
   D) Doxycycline
   E) Gentamicin

8. *Cystinuria is an inherited kidney and intestinal trans-epithelial transport defect for which amino acids?*

   A) Ornithine, leucine, alanine, cystine
   B) Ornithine, lysine, arginine, cystine
   C) Tyrosine, leucine, alanine, cystine
   D) Tyrosine, lysine, arginine, cystine
   E) Tyrosine, lysine, asparagine, cystine

9. *What do neutrophils produce in infected urine?*

   A) Leucocyte dehydrogenase
   B) Leucocyte esterase
   C) Leucocyte phosphatase
   D) Kallikreins
   E) Myeloperoxidase

10. *Which indicator dye is used on standard urine dipsticks to detect presence of protein in urine?*

   A) Hydroxyphenol
   B) Hydroxyphenylacetate
   C) Anthracene blue
   D) Tetrabromophenol
   E) Chromogen

11. *Where are Tamm–Horsfall proteins (involved in host defence mechanisms against UTI) made?*

    A) Bowman's capsule
    B) Collecting ducts
    C) Loop of Henle
    D) Adrenal gland
    E) Liver

12. *Which of the following antibiotics is not a bactericidal agent?*

    A) Cefalexin
    B) Penicillin
    C) Nitrofurantoin
    D) Gentamicin
    E) Trimethoprim

13. *Which of the following enzymes does trimethoprim inhibit?*

    A) Dihydropteroate synthase
    B) Topoisomerase II
    C) β-lactamase
    D) Dihydrofolate reductase
    E) DNA gyrase

14. *Which of the following antibiotics is most likely to be associated with the development of pulmonary fibrosis when used in low-dose continuous form for prophylaxis against rUTI?*

    A) Trimethoprim
    B) Cefalexin
    C) Nitrofurantoin
    D) Fosfomycin
    E) Sulfamethoxazole

15. *Which are the two most likely antibiotics you would choose to treat epididymitis in a patient who recently tested positive for chlamydia?*

    A) Doxycycline and azithromycin
    B) Doxycycline and ciprofloxacin
    C) Ciprofloxacin and azithromycin
    D) Ceftriaxone and ciprofloxacin
    E) Ceftriaxone and azithromycin

16. *A patient with emphysematous pyelonephritis is reported on the CT scan as having Class 2 Huang and Tseng grading. What does this mean?*

    A) Extension of gas into perinephric space
    B) Parenchymal gas only
    C) Gas in collecting system only
    D) Extension of gas into pararenal space
    E) Mild emphysematous pyelonephritis in single kidney

17. *Which of the following best describes a xanthoma?*

    A) Collection of xanthine crystals
    B) Collection of M2 macrophages
    C) Tumour of carbohydrate-rich monocytes
    D) Tumour of lipid poor macrophages
    E) Tumour of foam cells

18. *Which of the following is the intermediate snail host for S.haematobium?*

    A) Choanomphala
    B) Pfeifferi
    C) Oncomelania
    D) Biomphalaria
    E) Bulinus

19. *What is the correct dose of praziquantel to treat urinary schistosomiasis?*

    A) 10mg/kg
    B) 20mg/kg
    C) 40mg/kg
    D) 80mg/kg
    E) 160mg/kg

20. *Which of the following is the correct standard regimen for treating TB?*

    A) None of these
    B) 2 months (rifampicin, isoniazid, pyridoxine, ethambutol), then 4 months (isoniazid, rifampicin)
    C) 4 months (rifampicin, isoniazid, pyridoxine, ethambutol), then 2 months (isoniazid, rifampicin)
    D) 2 months (rifampicin, isoniazid, pyrazinamide, ethambutol), then 4 months (isoniazid, rifampicin)
    E) 4 months (rifampicin, isoniazid, pyrazinamide, ethambutol), then 2 months (isoniazid, rifampicin)

STATION 6
UROLOGICAL IMAGING & PRINCIPLES OF UROLOGICAL TECHNOLOGY

MEASUREMENT OF GFR

MEASUREMENT OF GFR

GFR is the volume of plasma filtered by the glomeruli in mL/minute.

Measured as clearance of any substance that is filtered but not actively secreted or reabsorbed by the tubules. Inulin is an ideal GFR marker but is difficult to assay in clinical practice.

Endogenous markers are used in daily practice; however, exogenous markers are used if more accurate measurements are required (see "Nuclear Medicine" section below).

GFR is proportional to body surface area and expressed as mL/min/1.73m2 ($1.73m^2$ is considered the average adult body surface area).

Normal values are generally > 90mL/min/1.73m^2.

CREATININE

Creatinine is primarily filtered at the glomerulus, its production is relatively stable and hence can be used as surrogate marker to estimate GFR (see Image 1).

Image 1 – Relationship between creatinine clearance and serum creatinine

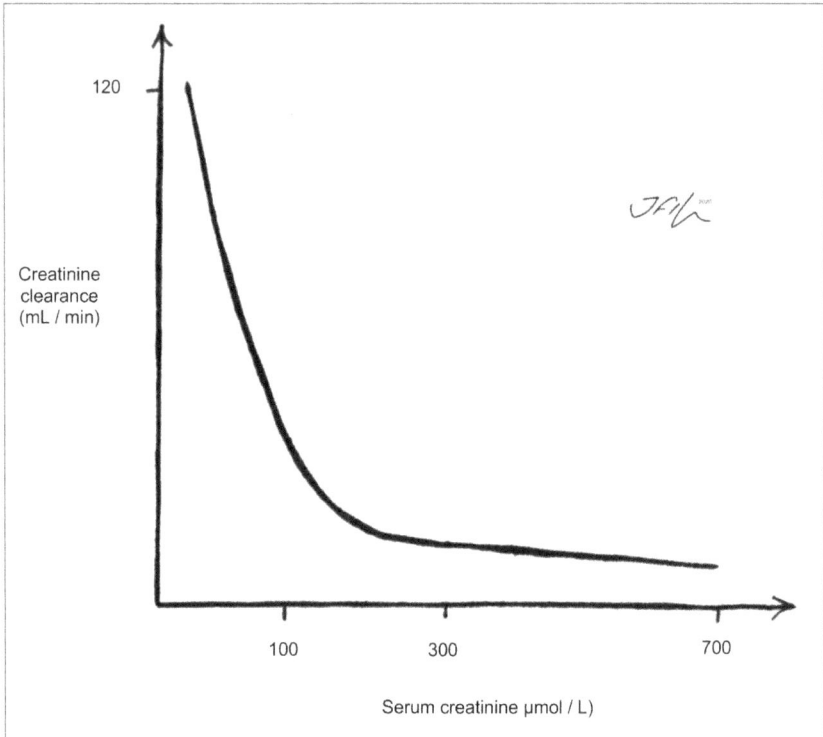

Image 1 suggests GFR calculation in relation to creatinine is less accurate as serum creatinine rises.

Creatinine tends to over-estimate GFR when function is normal.

Creatinine is affected by muscle mass and 10–20% is secreted by tubules.

Equations that can be used to estimate GFR include:

- *Cockcroft–Gault* formula – uses age, body mass and serum creatinine
- *MDRD* formula – uses age, gender, serum creatinine and Afro-Caribbean ethnicity (yes/no).

UROFLOWMETRY

Urinary flow-rate objective evaluation should be used as first-line investigation of male patients with voiding dysfunction.

Uroflowmetry is an assessment of flow; however, provides limited inference regarding detrusor function.

Patients being tested should have a normal desire to void and a voided volume ideally > 200mL.

Currently, there are three established mechanical means of measuring urinary flow – spinning disc, weight transduc.er and capacitance. [1]

Each system has a funnel to collect urine, a flow measurement device and a means of data recording.

1. *Rotating disc:*

   Urine is voided onto a disc which spins at constant speed – the power required to maintain this constant speed is proportional to the flow of urine opposing it.

2. *Weight transducer:*

   Relies on gravimetric principle as the weight of urine collected indicates the volume; by differentiation the flow rate can be calculated.

3. *Capacitance:*

   As the patient voids and thus the height of the column of urine increases, the electrical capacitance of a bimetallic strip mounted in the chamber changes.

Artefacts on Trace

- *Cough* – short sharp spike of increased flow
- *Valsalva* – wider increased flow spike
- *Cruising* – patient misdirecting urine flow, causes flow spike with decreased flow either side
- *Occlusion* – patients occludes urethra obliterating flow, increased flow on patient release
- *Knocking* – patient kicks device, high spike of flow which is very sharp and not physiological

PRINCIPLES OF RADIOLOGY

X-RAYS

XR are part of the spectrum of electromagnetic radiation, comprising of electric and magnetic waves travelling perpendicular to one another.

XR wavelength is shorter than that of visible light, in the order of 10^{-8} to 10^{-12}m.

Production of XR requires production of free electrons, which for purposes of clinical radiology occurs via heating a metal filament (the cathode) resulting in thermionic emission.

Electrons are accelerated in a vacuum toward a rotating metal anode where x-rays are produced.

XR beam is focused toward patient, placed between the XR source and a detector.

Tissues of different density cause attenuation of XR at different rates. Although XR attenuation is crucial to image formation, it is also a radiation dose to the patient.

XR KUB is readily available, easily interpreted and will reveal the majority of stones (60–90%); however, not uric acid, cystine (poorly) and indinavir.

Radiation Levels

Sievert – measure of health effect of low levels of radiation on the body (Sv unit is often too large for clinical use, so mSv used instead), intended to represent stochastic health risk (see below). [2]

Gray – 1Gy is radiation dose resulting in energy deposition of 1J/kg, used for higher doses of radiation that produce deterministic effects (see below) (e.g. dose of therapeutic radiotherapy).

Background radiation is 2–3mSv/year.

Table 1 – Common imaging with ionising radiation and their equivalent radiation dose

Imaging Technique	Approximate Radiation Dose (mSv)
CXR	0.02
XR KUB	0.5
IVU	1–2
CT KUB	4–5
CT urogram	10
DMSA	0.001–0.4
MAG3	2.6
PET	10

Protection From Radiation

Radiation obeys the inverse-square law (doubling your distance from the source quarters the radiation exposure) i.e. keep as great a distance away as possible.

Ionising radiation has two distinguishable types of effect on the body:

1. *Deterministic*, e.g. erythema, cataracts. There is a threshold dose below which no damage occurs. Side-effect severity depends on the dose of radiation, dose rate, and number of exposures. [3]

2. *Stochastic*, e.g. carcinogenesis and mutagenesis. No threshold dose; even a single exposure can result in damage. Frequency of stochastic effects increases with increasing dose, but their severity does not. They occur on random basis and are a mutation effect.

CONTRAST AGENTS

Contrast agents are a heterogeneous group of pharmaceuticals used during radiological procedures to enhance tissue definition.

Three groups of intravenous contrast agents are broadly available – iodinated agents, gadolinium and microbubble particles.

IODINATED AGENTS

Formed from organic acid salts of iodine.

The relatively high molecular weight of iodine I127 makes it radio-opaque.

When injected intravenously, iodinated agents are rapidly eliminated by renal excretion.

Iodinated agents are safe with generally low rates of adverse reaction (0.15%) e.g. nausea and vomiting, urticaria, skin rash.

Severe reactions are rare (< 0.01%) and include bronchospasm, laryngeal oedema and anaphylaxis (death rate estimated 1 in 100,000).

Contrast-induced nephropathy is a concern with iodinated agents.

The single most effective method to reduce risk of renal injury due to IV contrast is aggressive IV hydration before and after the contrast is administered for the scan.

The American College of Radiology defines post-contrast AKI as $\geq 1.5x$ increase in creatinine from baseline within 48–72 hours. [4]

There is no absolute GFR value below which contrast cannot be given – this decision will vary between radiologists and on a case-by-case basis.

A commonly applied rationale is generally:

- GFR > 30 – proceed
- GFR 15–30 – equivocal (consider admission for pre- and post-contrast IV hydration)
- GFR < 15 – do not proceed unless dialysis available.

Patients who have low GFR and take metformin must pause this the day before their scan, withhold 48 hours after the scan, re-start only provided GFR has not declined.

Poor metformin clearance may cause lactic acidosis.

Contraindications

The Royal College of Radiologists states that increased risk of adverse reactions may be seen in: [5]

- Renal impairment
- Previous adverse reaction
- Asthma (avoid if patient is wheezy)
- Diabetes and metformin therapy
- Pregnancy.

GADOLINIUM

The most widely used contrast agents for MR imaging are chelates of gadolinium.

Adverse reactions are low (0.04%) and serious anaphylactic reaction extremely rare.

Nephrogenic systemic fibrosis is a potentially fatal condition characterised by development of fibrotic tissue in skin and muscles due to accumulation of gadolinium in these tissues. [6]

There is no consistently successful treatment for nephrogenic systemic fibrosis.

MICROBUBBLES

Microbubbles are IV contrast agents used in contrast-enhanced US.

They consist of a gas surrounded by a lipid or polymer shell, ranging 2–10μ in size.

Microbubbles have a high degree of echogenicity, much greater than surrounding soft tissues of the body, making it ideal to visualise blood perfusion in organs.

DEXA SCAN

DEXA scans are used to estimate BMD, which is key to diagnose osteoporosis/osteopaenia.

DEXA works by emitting low-dose XR beam with two distinct energy peaks (one absorbed by soft tissue and the other by bone); absorption subtraction allows for BMD calculation.

Patient is supine, clothed (however, no garments with metal), the scan takes ~5 minutes.

BMD score is compared with sex-matched individuals to give WHO-defined T-score which is based on the number of standard deviations from a normal healthy adult:

- More than 2.5 SD below normal is osteoporosis (i.e. -2.5 or less)
- 1 to 2.5 SD below normal is osteopaenia (i.e. -1.5 to -2.5)
- Within 1 SD is normal (i.e. -1 to +1).

Z-score is comparison of patient's BMD with matched age and gender reference values.

Z-scores are used in determining osteoporosis in young men, premenopausal women, children.

DEXA should be offered to men starting long-term ADT in prostate cancer to provide a baseline BMD at diagnosis (EAU 2024). [7]

Osteoporosis in prostate cancer should be prevented with weight optimisation, regular exercise and ensuring vitamin D and calcium are within recommended levels.

ULTRASONOGRAPHY

US waves are produced by the application of a voltage across a piezoelectric crystal which deforms, converting electrical energy into sound energy.

US waves are propagated through body tissues at speeds which vary according to tissue composition.

When US hits interface between tissues it may be transmitted, refracted, absorbed or reflected.

US coupling gel is used to reduce the attenuation occurring at skin interface with probe.

A proportion of the reflected US waves will pass back to the transducer where the piezoelectric process is reversed; sound is converted to an electrical impulse which generates the image.

The shades of grey on the image are determined by the strength of returning US waves e.g. stones are white (high echogenicity), soft tumour is grey, water is black.

The processes of absorption, refraction and reflection are collectively termed *attenuation*.

Lower frequencies are used to look at deeper tissues (attenuation greater at higher frequencies).

Applications within Urology

The following frequencies are used to visualise the below areas via US:

- Prostate TRUS: 6–10MHz (prostate is close to probe)
- Abdominal US: 3.5MHz
- Testicular US: 7–12MHz.

Therapeutic applications of ultrasonography include ESWL and HIFU.

HIFU uses a frequency of 1–3.5MHz focused to reach high intensity in thermal target area (a cooling balloon protects the rectal mucosa) to reach ≤ 90°C.

Tissue damage occurs by coagulative necrosis – thermal injury and cavitation (microbubble formation and collapse). [8]

HIFU not currently recommended by NICE as a treatment for prostate cancer, other than in the context of controlled clinical trials.

Doppler Ultrasound

Doppler principle is the change in the frequency of a wave in relation to an observer who is moving relative to the source.

If the frequency of the transmitted beam is known and the frequency of the reflected sound is measured, the velocity can be calculated.

Doppler US can be used to measure blood flow (US waves bounce off red blood cells).

MAGNETIC RESONANCE IMAGING

Protons of hydrogen atoms usually spin in random fashion.

Upon entering an MRI scanner they align with the magnetic field in the longitudinal plane and produce a secondary spin (precession).

When radio-frequency pulse is applied, the nuclei receive energy to move out of alignment and into the transverse plane.

When this pulse is removed the atoms release their energy in 2 ways:

- T1 relaxation: energy released back into surroundings (realign back to longitudinal plane)
- T2 decay: energy loss between adjacent nuclei.

The release of energy is picked up as an electrical voltage by a receiver coil (MR signal).

MpMRI combines anatomical sequences (T1 and T2) with functional sequences (DWI, DCE, ADC) to improve accuracy of prostate cancer diagnosis.

T1 Image

T1 relaxation occurs more rapidly in fat (large molecules give energy back to environment quicker).

Fat appears very bright, fluid remains dark, such that these scans are excellent for viewing anatomy due to the good tissue differentiation.

T2 Image

T2 decay occurs more slowly in water, resulting in higher signal.

Water has a very bright signal on these images, producing a scan which is more useful for revealing pathology (water appears white).

Prostate cancer appears dark/black in prostate cancer.

| VIVA | If you are shown an MRI in the FRCS (Urol) viva and you are unsure as to the type of image it is, look at the bladder contents and/or CSF – if these are bright/white, image is T2 sequence.

Diffusion Weighting

DW-MRI imaging exploits the random motion of water molecules (*"Brownian motion"*).

This free movement of water is restricted in the body by boundaries formed by cell membranes.

Tissues typically demonstrating restricted diffusion include cancer, oedema, fibrosis and abscess.

Densely packed prostate cancer cells display restricted diffusion on MRI compared to normal adjacent peripheral zone tissue cells.

Prostate cancer appears brighter than normal peripheral zone tissue on DW-MRI.

Dynamic Contrast Enhancement

DCE measures blood flow in/out of prostate tissue.

In prostate cancer there is rapid wash-in/-out, and therefore will show early enhancement.

Apparent Diffusion Coefficient

The impedance of DWI water molecules can be quantified with an ADC value, which is calculated by software and displayed as a parametric map (prostate cancer appears darker).

| VIVA | The most likely discussions or images pertaining to MRI scans in your FRCS (Urol) viva are going to be around mpMRI of the prostate. I would therefore recommend spending some time learning about these in more detail and practising the very basics of how to interpret them.

CONTRAINDICATIONS

Strong magnetic fields around MRI scanner ensure that some special precautions are necessary.

Contraindications to MRI which must be always cross-checked with attending radiographers include:

- Metallic foreign bodies, e.g. metal in eyes from welding
- Cardiac pacemakers (some are MRI compatible), cardiac devices, SNM devices
- Ferrous containing aneurysm coils.

COMPUTED TOMOGRAPHY

XR are produced when fast-moving electrons are stopped suddenly by impact on metal target.

The kinetic energy of the electrons is converted into XR (1%) and heat (99%).

An XR tube consists of two electrodes in a vacuum; a negative (cathode) and a positive (anode) electrode; along with a smooth flat metal target.

The cathode tungsten filament is heated and emits electrons by the process of thermionic emission.

The electrons are attracted and travel to the positive anode.

Each electron arrives at the target surface with a kinetic energy equivalent to the voltage (kV).

XR may be:

- *Transmitted:* pass through tissues unaffected
- *Absorbed:* transfer to the tissue some or all of their energy
- *Scattered:* diverted in a new direction, with or without loss of energy.

Attenuation is the reduction in intensity of the primary XR beam as it passes through a medium.

(Attenuation = Absorption + Scatter)

In CT, the XR beams are attenuated as they pass through the patient; detectors around the patient measure XR transmission many times from different directions as gantry rotates 360°.

CT image is reconstructed, where transmitted XR are measured and assigned to each pixel according to the degree of attenuation.

Hounsfield scale is used as a quantitative scale to describe radiodensity:

- Water is assigned value of 0
- Lowest end of the scale is -1,000HU for air
- Hard stones exceed +1,000HU.

CT UROGRAM

CTU protocols vary between Trusts and radiologists; however, a commonly used sequence includes:

- Initial non-contrast phase (plain CT KUB)
- Arterial phase – 20s (maximal enhancement of abdominal and renal vessels)
- Nephrographic phase – 70–90s (assess enhancement)
- Urographic phase – 5–10 minutes (pelvi-calyceal system, ureters, bladder).

Split-bolus technique can be used to reduce the radiation dose given to the patient:

- Initial non-contrast phase
- Administer 50% of the IV contrast and wait 7–8 minutes
- Then give remaining 50% of IV contrast
- CT is then performed after 60s to combine both urographic and nephrographic phases.

NUCLEAR MEDICINE

Nuclear medicine scans rely on emission radiography – providing functional information by injecting a radioactive agent (e.g. 99mTc) which is attached/chelated to a metabolite (e.g. MAG3).

MAG3 RENOGRAM

MAG3 is a renally excreted compound, cleared mostly by proximal tubular extraction which secretes it into the tubular lumen, as well as partly by glomerular filtration.

The renogram is achieved by chelation of MAG3 with 99mTc.

MAG3 renogram is a dynamic scan producing a video; images are extracted as a series of still photos.

MAG3 renogram is most useful when there is concern regarding upper-tract obstruction (e.g. PUJO) and it can also estimate split differential kidney function.

Renal glomeruli/tubules take $\geq$ 3 months to mature after birth – hence the recommendation that isotope renograms only be performed after this age has been reached.

The *diuresis renogram* is a variant of the standard renogram in which the urine flow rate is increased by administration of an IV diuretic (e.g. furosemide).

The diuretic response is proportional to the underlying renal function, therefore MAG3 should be interpreted with caution or indeed not performed at all in those with eGFR < 15mL/min.

Radioisotope

The most commonly used radioisotope is metastable technetium-99 (99mTc).

The half-life of 99mTc is 6 hours. [9]

Approximately 90% of 99mTc MAG3 is cleared in the urine by tubular secretion and 10% by glomerular filtration (furosemide is given to ensure kidneys are maximally diuresing).

^{99m}Tc decays by emission of gamma rays only (not α or β).

^{99m}Tc is available from a generator which provides a supply from the decay of longer-lived parent ^{99}Mo.

MAG3 Technique

The patient should be well-hydrated prior to the test.

Furosemide's maximal effect seen after ~20 minutes – used to be given 20 minutes after isotope (F+20 study) but this led to obstruction noted later in study and more chance of equivocal result.

Furosemide given 15 minutes prior to isotope injection (F-15 study) is now more commonly used.

Patient is either seated with back to gamma camera or supine with camera underneath.

After the isotope is injected the gamma camera starts immediately:

- Dynamic images taken every 2 seconds for one minute
- Then every 20 seconds for 30–40 minutes
- Patient asked to void at end of study and post-void image taken.

MAG3 Interpretation

On still images of dynamic series, regions of interest are drawn around each kidney.

Activity/time curves are created showing how activity in each region of interest changes with time, and a background curve is used to subtract background contribution from each kidney curve.

The resulting curve is a renogram.

The relative function of each kidney is calculated from the uptake phase (1–3 minutes).

MAG3 Phases

The study begins with the *vascular* phase:

- Occurs within first few seconds after isotope injection
- Represents rapid flow of isotope to the kidney
- Most of isotope is not extracted and remains in blood in kidney
- This phase should be removed from the renogram curve, which should rise smoothly.

From 1 minute onwards, renogram curve rises at rate proportional to kidney function (*uptake* phase).

From 3 minutes onwards, renogram curve may peak and begin to fall (*elimination* phase):

- This is a balance between elimination and uptake
- Rising curve means uptake exceeds elimination (falling curve implies the reverse).

- *Type I* – normal renal uptake and drainage
- *Type II* – obstructed pattern – no response to diuretic, curve rises or remains high
- *Type IIIa* – normal drainage but from hypotonic renal pelvis, falls rapidly after furosemide
- *Type IIIb* – equivocal, rises rapidly but neither falls nor rises after furosemide – this requires further evaluation, could be partial ureteric obstruction or impaired renal function
- *Type IV* (*Homsy's sign*) – furosemide causes transient response appearing decompensated at high flow suggesting likely obstruction; (F-15) is required to confirm

VIVA You may be asked to draw and/or interpret F+20 diuresis renogram curves (O'Reilly's curves) for the FRCS (Urol) viva. I recommend you practise drawing them until you can reproduce them comfortably and quickly (Figure 1).

Figure 1 – Diuresis renogram curves for F+20

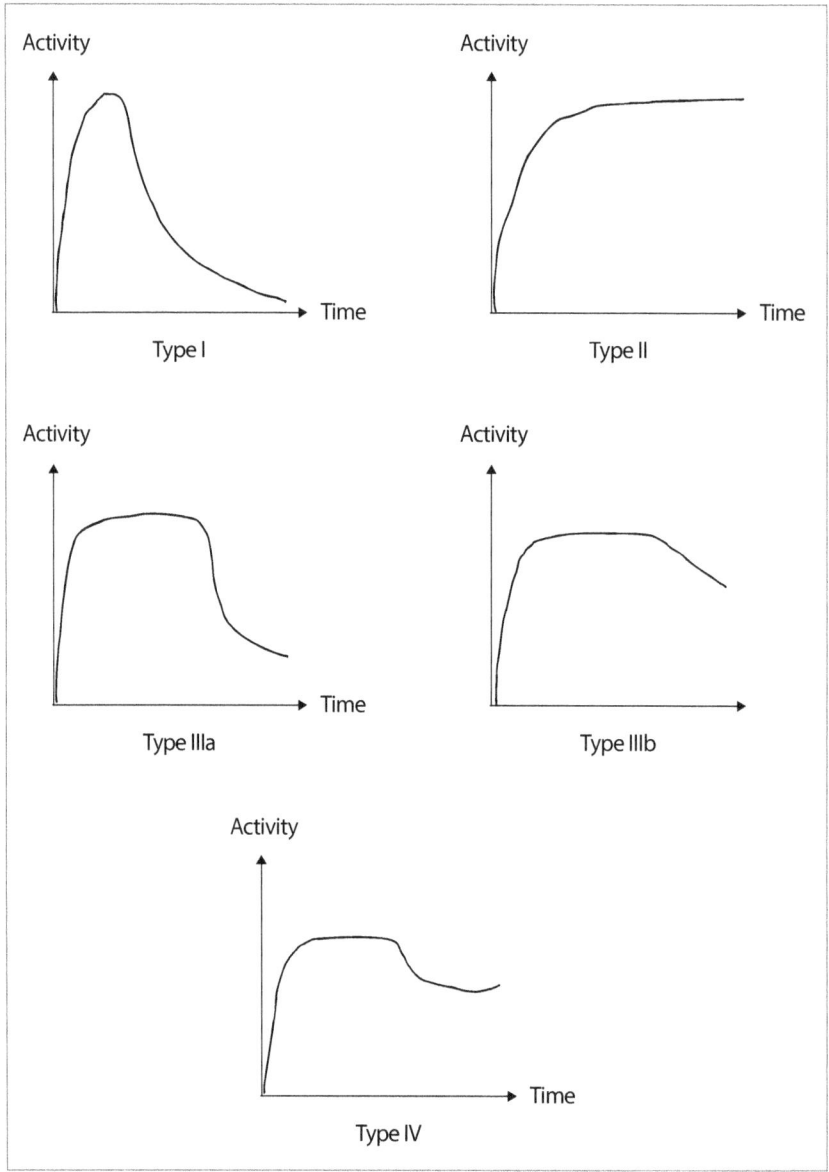

Whitaker Test

The Whitaker test is a mostly academic investigation for equivocal ureteric obstruction (e.g. Type IIIb curve) rarely performed in modern practice (F-15 phase could be tried first).

It is an invasive test requiring percutaneous access tube to the renal pelvis and a urethral catheter. [10]

Saline is infused at 10mL/min via renal pelvis and pressure difference is measured on the manometers on the renal tube and urethral catheter: [11]

- Pressure difference > 22cm H_2O = ureteric obstruction
- Pressure difference 15–22cm H_2O = equivocal
- Pressure difference < 15cm H_2O = obstructed.

DMSA SCAN

DMSA scan is a static nuclear medicine study – producing a still image.

DMSA is radiolabelled with 99mTc, whose radioactivity can be measured.

DMSA is a protein actively extracted and bound by functioning renal tubules, very little is filtered and it is not secreted.

Kidney detail/resolution in DMSA scans is much more detailed than those seen in MAG3 renograms, for example being able to reveal cortical defects in acute pyelonephritis or renal scarring.

DMSA scans also give good detail in duplex kidneys showing the function of each moiety.

DMSA scans are most useful, therefore, when detailed information is required about the kidney and there is no concern regarding underlying renal obstruction.

Active infection may distort images – wait ≥ 6 weeks after pyelonephritis resolution before scanning.

DMSA Technique

The patient must wait 2–4 hours after the DMSA injection to allow sufficient time for cortical uptake to take place prior to imaging being undertaken.

Patient is then positioned supine on couch.

Static views of kidney are taken from different projections (e.g. anterior, posterior, oblique).

PET SCAN

PET is a form of nuclear medicine imaging which uses positron-emitting radionuclides rather than the gamma-emitting radionuclides used in renography.

There are several radionuclides suitable for PET imaging – choice will depend on half-life of agent.

Most common radiotracer used in general clinical practice is 18F-labelled FDG:

- Analogue of glucose
- More glucose required by anaerobic glycolysis in cancers than aerobic in normal tissue
- Pronounced FDG uptake seen within cancerous tissue.

Increased FDG uptake is not specific to glucose metabolism within tumours, it can be raised in areas of infection/inflammation, due to accumulation in macrophages/neutrophils.

Choline (11C) and PSMA PET are options for prostate cancer investigations.

PET Technique

Radiotracer is injected into patient and processed by body, accumulating in the tissue of interest.

When the tracer decays it emits a positron which should annihilate with a nearby electron to produce two back-to-back photons.

This encounter occurs along *"line of response"* – millions of these are recorded in typical PET scan and reconstructed to map out 3D distribution of radionuclide within body.

PET is often combined with CT allowing for information on tissue function to be superimposed onto structural information from the CT.

Urological Applications

The following are some examples of practical application of PET in urological practice:

- *Prostate cancer*, to investigate biochemical relapse after RP or RTx (^{11}C)
- *Testicular cancer*, for persisting nodal mass > 3cm in seminomatous GCT (^{18}FDG)
- *Penile cancer*, for assessment of nodal disease in advanced cases.

FDG cannot be used in urothelial cancers as it is renally excreted and accumulates in urinary tract.

PSMA scan is labelled with gallium (^{68}Ga) and is more expensive than standard ^{11}C PET as the radioisotope is less stable and cannot be stored.

PSMA is the imaging modality of choice to detect biochemical relapse of prostate cancer at low PSA levels (e.g. < 0.5ng/mL) as it has the highest sensitivity and is superior to 11C PET.

EAU 2024 recommends PSMA PET be offered to men with persistent PSA > 0.2ng/mL after radical treatment if available. [7]

If PSMA PET unavailable, 11C PET can be used, but PSA threshold likely to be higher (e.g. > 1.0ng/mL).

Single-photon Emission Computed Tomography

SPECT is similar to conventional PET except SPECT measures gamma radiation emitted directly (whereas PET measures positrons that have annihilated electrons nearby, emitting photons).

SPECT relies on radioisotope (e.g. gallium) attached to a specific ligand, whose properties bind it to a certain type of tissue.

Gamma camera rotates around patient collecting images which are reconstructed to form a 3D image.

RADIOISOTOPE MEASUREMENT OF GFR

GFR can be measured by blood clearance of any tracer which is cleared through kidneys solely by glomerular filtration.

Nuclear medicine is ideal because it uses minute quantities of tracer radioisotope that do not disturb kidney function and give a very low radiation dose.

The method involves blood sampling alone and so is helpful when urine collection is difficult.

More accurate than eGFR, which is based on a serum creatinine measurement in isolation.

Radioisotope measurement of GFR only evaluates total renal clearance, therefore individual differential kidney clearance can only be inferred in combination with either MAG3 or DMSA.

51Cr EDTA or 99mTc DTPA are radionuclides that can be used (solely cleared by glomerular filtration).

Study Technique

Patient is injected with selected radioisotope.

Blood samples are taken from opposite arm at 2, 3, 4 and 5 hours after injection.

Samples are centrifuged to yield plasma which is then measured for radioactivity – a graph is plotted of plasma counts vs. time since injection.

The graph line is extrapolated back to time zero.

The slope determines the clearance rate. [12]

NUCLEAR BONE SCAN

A nuclear medicine bone scan is used for detecting areas of abnormal bone metabolism.

Indicated for identifying presence or progression of bone metastases in cancer staging investigations.

MDP or HDP (bisphosphonate derivatives) are radiolabelled with 99mTc for use in bone scans.

These scans will show areas of normal vs. abnormal metabolism and are very sensitive.

They are also excreted in the urine, so kidneys/bladder will also be seen on the image (i.e. hydronephrosis or urinary retention may be incidentally noted).

Typical radiation dose is 4–6mSv.

Study Technique

Three hours after injection, images showing bone metabolism are acquired in a variety of ways:

- Whole-body image: camera slowly moves along length of patient taking about 20 minutes to produce a whole-body scan
- SPECT: gamma camera rotates all the way round the patient taking images from many angles (20 minutes) which are then reconstructed.

The bone scan has 3 phases:

- Flow phase: within 60 seconds
- Blood pool phase: within 5 minutes
- Delayed phase: 2–4 hours.

Hot spots are areas of increased uptake, indicating increased bone metabolism.

These are not specific to metastases and may be seen in fractures, Paget's and degeneration.

Superscan implies heavy metastatic infiltration such that soft-tissue/urinary-tract uptake is minimal.

| VIVA | If you are shown a bone scan in your FRCS (Urol) viva, be aware that on a metastatic superscan if the involvement is sufficiently uniform, the scan may appear deceptively normal. Therefore carefully correlate what you are seeing to the clinical scenario you have been presented with. |

OPTICS, SCOPES AND ACCESSORIES

HOPKINS ROD-LENS SYSTEM

This involves a series of long glass rods in a metal cylinder separated by short airspaces.

Light is transmitted by optic-fibre bundles running from external light source (usually halogen light which is yellow, hence the need for white balancing).

The advantages of the Hopkins rod-lens system include:

- Superior light passage and image quality
- Reduced diameter of instrument
- Colour reproduction.

This particular type of lens is only used in rigid cystoscopes.

OPTIC FIBRES

Optic fibres are flexible glass (or plastic) fibres that allow light to pass through them via a process called total internal reflection.

Fibres are grouped together in parallel fashion and protected by external plastic sleeves.

They are used for rigid/flexible URS.

Optic fibres within urology have two main uses:

- Transmission of light from external source to endoscope: the fibres need not be coherent
- Transmission of images: this relies on coherent bundles of optic fibres.

The distal tip objective lens can be angled to give an oblique view – e.g. 12°, 30°, 70°.

Digital scopes utilise a chip at the distal end of the scope which transmits a digital image.

SCOPES

The French gauge (Fr) was developed by Charriere – corresponds to 3x the diameter (in mm) – e.g. 21Fr cystoscope sheath has an external diameter of 7mm.

Cystoscopes

Adult cystoscope sheaths are generally between 17–25Fr (approximately 30cm long).

These have a telescope inside, a bridge/working element and an outer sheath.

Cystoscopes available in different angles and are marked accordingly with a coloured cuff:

- 0° – green
- 30° – red
- 70° – yellow.

Resectoscopes are larger (e.g. 26–28Fr).

A *leak test* should be undertaken prior to use and before cleaning the scope – this is to check whether fluid is entering the scope.

Attach a manometer to the scope and inflate – the pressure should be maintained; if it is not, this suggests a leak is present and the scope should be sent for repair.

Semi-rigid URS

Rigid URS scopes use fibre-optics for image transmission, not the rod-lens system.

The instrument length is approximately 34cm long.

The tip of the instrument is 7–10Fr:

- One working channel implies 3.4Fr
- If two channels are present, they are approximately 2.3Fr each.

Flexible URS

Length may vary between 70–80cm.

Distal end of the instrument is 5.4Fr (working channels 3.6Fr approximately), which permits passage of instruments such as baskets or LASER fibres.

Flexible URS may be passed into kidney via access sheaths.

Disposable scopes are digital, single-use and have no need for white balancing.

Access Sheath

Access sheaths are used to establish a conduit during endo-urological procedures, to facilitate the repeated passage of instruments to the upper tract.

Access sheaths can be 40–45cm in length and 10–14Fr.

Access sheaths are hydrophilic (i.e. dampen before use); consist of an internal obturator and an outer sheath; lumen is made of PTFE; distal tip starts at 6Fr and tapers wider.

They decrease intra-renal pressure during URS.

ENDOSCOPIC INSTRUMENTS

Albarran bridge

Albarran lever/bridge is required for the endoscopic deflection of peripheral instruments.

You must ensure the level is flat to the scope when inserting this into urethra, otherwise the lever can injure the urethral lining and cause false passages.

Alligator and Biopsy Forceps

These have to be completely outside the working channel, otherwise the hinge mechanism will not be able to open properly.

Stone Cone

Device which can be deployed within the ureter, distal to the stone, to prevent proximal migration of fragments during intra-corporeal lithotripsy.

Nitinol inner core with PTFE outer layer.

Baskets

There are many different baskets available for use in endo-urology.

Most have a straight tip guide, placed beyond the stone providing greater stability when in use.

The handles of all modern baskets can be dismantled to allow backward removal of the URS whilst basket remains in place.

This is invaluable when the basket and stone gets trapped in the ureter, permitting removal of the scope and reinsertion alongside the basket.

Wires

Guidewires in the ureter are placed for access, security and increasing stability of the ureter.

The diameter is 0.035in or 0.038in (typical length 150cm).

Important variable characteristics of wires include tip shape, shaft rigidity, torque (property that allows movement at one end to be transmitted to distal end) and surface resistance.

Guidewire selection depends on the circumstances demanded by the procedure.

Access to the ureter is often achieved via sensor wire:

- Hydrophilic flexible tip to minimise trauma (tungsten filled for fluoroscopic visualisation)
- *Nitinol* (nickel–titanium alloy) + stainless-steel core
- PTFE coating to offer smooth wire surface.

Guidewires with higher rigidity are chosen when greater stability needed e.g. Amplatz super-stiff:

- Large inner stainless-steel core
- PTFE coating for smoothness.

In difficult ureteric navigation, a slippery hydrophilic guidewire (e.g. Terumo®) can be used:

- Nitinol core covered with polyurethane containing tungsten
- Hydrophilic polymer coating.

Ureteric Catheter

Ureteric catheters are approximately 6Fr in size with a length of 70cm and are PTFE coated.

Most have 1cm markings along the length.

In urological practice they can be:

- Introduced into the ureteric orifice to perform retrograde studies
- Used to help ureteric orifice cannulation with guidewires (e.g. tight or difficult angle)
- Left in situ in the ureter as a short-term measure of protecting ureteric patency (e.g. post-URS).

STENTS AND CATHETERS

URETERIC STENTS

Most urine drains around stents by *coaptive peristalsis* rather than through the central lumen, except at points of complete obstruction where it passes through side holes into the lumen.

Different materials can be used to make stents; most of these are polymers.

The presence of silicone increases rigidity and allows a lifetime of ≤ 12 months.

Implanted plastic tubes will cause production of sialomucins dependent upon their composition.

All tubes in the urinary tract will develop a *biofilm* and become encrusted with constituents of urine, and will encrust more rapidly in stone former's or pregnant patient urine.

Foreign bodies should remain in situ for shortest time possible in stone formers, as encrustation starts within days of implantation and may occlude the stent lumen within a week.

All plastic stents require insertion over a guidewire under radiological control.

The whole length of a double-J stent has small holes drilled in it to facilitate drainage.

Double-J stents are 18–30cm long (pre-formed coil at each end) and 4.7–8Fr.

Stents may be coated with hydrophilic Teflon or antibacterial coatings to make insertion easier or to try to reduce bacterial adherence and encrustation.

Radio-opacity of stents is increased by coating them with metals such as bismuth and barium.

Indications for Stenting

Emergency indications for ureteric stenting include:

- Relief of ureteric obstruction
- Following trauma to the ureter
- Drainage of acutely infected kidney.

Elective indications for ureteric stenting include:

- Protection of anastomosis (e.g. pyeloplasty, ureteric reimplantation)
- Pre-operatively to aid identification of the ureter
- To protect drainage following endo-urological stone procedures.

Metallic Stents

Metallic ureteric stents are used mainly in management of ureteric strictures.

The *Memokath* stent is made of nitinol (nickel-titanium memory-shape alloy).

Not widely used in clinical practice due to challenges such as encrustation and difficult exchanges.

Resonance® stents are made of metallic alloy, they can stay longer in situ and are inserted through an 8Fr outer sheath, purported to be more resistant to extrinsic ureteric obstruction.

Multi-length Stent

Some stents have a multi-length coil on either end, which means that the stent uncoils in capacious areas such as renal pelvis or bladder.

Main advantage is that fewer lengths of stent are needed to be kept in stock.

Polaris™ stents have a double coil in bladder to reduce stent symptoms – not often used.

PROSTATIC/URETHRAL STENTS

These were developed to treat men with recurrent urethral strictures, BOO unfit for surgical intervention or, rarely, for treating DetSD.

They are not routinely used in practice anymore.

Reasons for their lack of establishment in urological practice include:

- Advances in minimally invasive BOO surgery techniques
- Stent migration resulting in urinary retention
- Stent encrustation, blockage and infection.

URINARY CATHETERS

Urinary catheters are inserted for three main reasons:

- Drainage of urine for diagnostic or therapeutic intent
- Access to flush intra-vesical medications (e.g. BCG, MMC)
- Diagnostic studies (e.g. urethrogram, cystogram).

The variables when describing a urinary catheter may include:

- *Size:* expressed in French scale (Charriere gauge)
- *Channels:* usually 2- or 3-way
- *Tip design:* Foley (standard), Tiemann (curve tip), Coude (curve tip)
- *Materials:* silicone (long term ≤ 3 months) or PTFE/latex (short term ≤ 28 days).

Catheter ring colours include 12F (white), 14F (green), 16F (orange), 18F (red).

Catheter bypassing is distressing and difficult to manage – anticholinergics, diazepam and reducing balloon size may all be tried.

All catheterised patients eventually develop bacteriuria (mostly within 28 days) – treat only if systemic symptoms; the catheter in the unwell patient will have biofilm on it and needs replacing.

Asymptomatic catheter-associated bacteriuria should not be treated (EAU 2024). [13]

If catheter-related UTI is suspected, replace catheter before initiating antimicrobial therapy (EAU 2024).

Biofilm Formation

A biofilm is a consortium of micro-organisms in which cells stick to each other and surface.

This confers a survival advantage to the microbes such that infections are resistant to antibiotics. [14]

There are 5 stages to biofilm formation:

1. Adhesion to surface
2. Aggregation
3. Biofilm formation
4. 3-dimensional growth
5. Micro-organism release to colonise other surfaces.

LITHOTRIPSY

EXTRA-CORPOREAL LITHOTRIPSY

The components of an ESWL machine include:

1. *Energy source* – can be electrohydraulic, electromagnetic, piezoelectric – the resulting shockwave produced from all these sources is the same

2. *Coupling mechanism* – a gel- or water-filled cushion is used to transmit the energy

3. *Imaging* – US or fluoroscopy can be used to localise the stone

4. *Focusing system* – required to concentrate energy on stone, elliptical (electrohydraulic ESWL), hemi-spherical (piezoelectric ESWL), cylindrical reflector (electromagnetic ESWL).

Electrohydraulic ESWL

Electrohydraulic lithotripters were the earliest extra-corporeal devices developed.

They produce a spark between two electrodes under water resulting in rapid expansion and collapse of gas bubbles and subsequent energy transmission (see Image 2).

Example of electrohydraulic lithotripter is Dornier HM3.

Electromagnetic ESWL

Electromagnetic lithotripters rely on a cylindrical electromagnetic source – a coil of wire in close proximity to a thin metal membrane with water on the other side.

Current passes through the coil which repulses the metal membrane and generates a pressure pulse in water – this is focused by an acoustic lens (see Image 2).

One of the more commonly used machines in routine practice, for example, is the Storz MODULITH®.

Piezoelectric ESWL

Piezoelectric materials consist of ceramic or crystal elements that produce an electrical discharge under stress or tension.

Energy transmission is produced via movement of the source when electricity is passed through it.

Piezoelectric elements are placed on a concave surface which focuses the waves onto the stone (see Image 2).

An example of a piezoelectric lithotripter is the Richard Wolf PiezoLith 3000.

Image 2 – Diagrammatic representation of the 3 types of ESWL

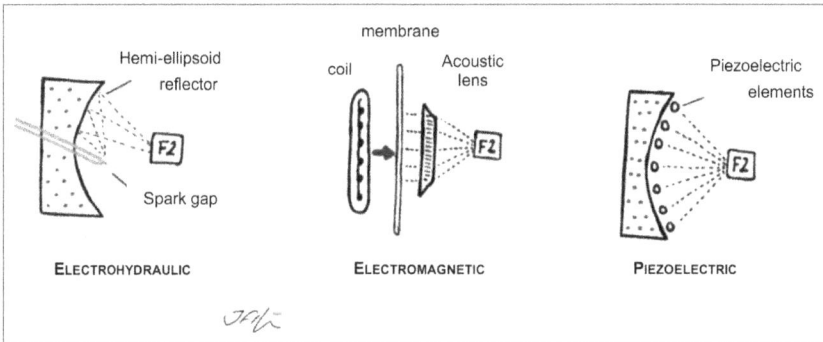

SHOCKWAVE PHASES

The acoustic shockwave has two main phases (Image 3):

- First a short positive phase, causing erosion and entry and exit points of the stone, and internal shattering due to compressive effects of the wave

- Then a longer negative pressure phase which results in formation of microbubbles, which collapse and form micro-jets which further erode the stone.

VIVA You may be asked to draw an acoustic shockwave graph in your FRCS (Urol) viva. Please ensure you can reproduce this seamlessly. You should also know how to label the graph axes and add typical numerical values of the pressures.

Image 3 – Waveform of shockwave

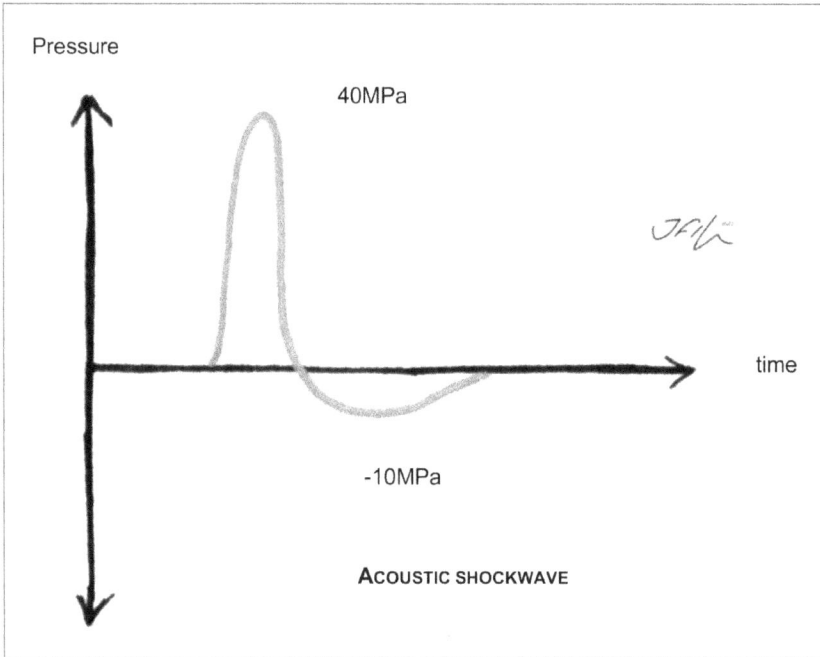

INTRA-CORPOREAL LITHOTRIPSY

Ultrasonic Lithotripsy

US waves produced by a generator are transmitted down a hollow probe resulting in vibration of the probe tip, which will drill/fragment stones when in contact with them.

Not for use in ureter as tip vibration causes heat production which may result in perforation.

Ballistic Lithotripsy

Forward momentum of metal rod placed in contact with stone surface.

Swiss LithoClast™ uses a controlled burst of compressed air to move as a projectile. Has tendency to move stones forward and can only be used in rigid scope.

Swiss LithoClast™ Master combines US with ballistics and suction, often used in PCNL.

LASER LITHOTRIPSY

LASER is created by applying energy to a lasing medium, where a photon is released from an atom within the medium, and further collides with excited atoms to release more photons.

This process is called spontaneous emission.

The most commonly used LASER is the holmium: yttrium-aluminium-garnet (Ho:YAG).

Ho:YAG wavelength is 2,140nm.

Fibre sizes commonly used are 200µm (kidney), 365µm (ureter) and 500µm (bladder).

LASER fibres are made of silica/silicon dioxide (i.e. glass).

Characteristics of LASER light include:

- *Mono-chromatic* (single colour) defined by its wavelength
- *Collimated* (travel in parallel beam) guided through optical fibres focused on small spot
- *Coherent* (waves are in phase).

Tissue is affected by LASER energy by absorbing light and converting it to thermal energy.

It will target a tissue that absorbs the particular wavelength it is set at.

LASER energy breaks stones by:

- Vaporisation – temperatures reach > 100°C
- Photo-acoustic mechanism – whereby pulsed LASER forms plasma bubbles which expand and collapse generating a shockwave.

LASER effects are limited to ≤ 1mm from fibre tip, hence risk of urothelial injury is minimised.

The different types and applications of LASER within urology are shown in Table 2.

Table 2 – LASERs used in urology and their properties [15]

Active Crystal	Abbreviation	Wavelength (nm)	Applications	Penetration (mm)
Holmium	Ho:YAG	2,140	HoLEP, ablation of TCC Stone fragmentation	0.4
Neodynium	Nd:YAG	1,064	Ablation of TCC Coagulation of prostate tissue	10
Kalium titanyl phosphate (Greenlight)	KTP:Nd:YAG	532	Absorbed by haemoglobin, used to vaporise prostate tissue	0.8
Lithium borate (Greenlight)	LBO:Nd:YAG	532	Absorbed by haemoglobin, used to vaporise prostate tissue	0.8
Thulium	Tm:YAG	2,013	Ablation of TCC Vaporisation of prostate	0.25

LASER Safety

The main risks of LASER are burns and injuries to the eye.

Different LASERs pose different risks e.g. Nd:YAG has penetration depth of 10mm and can cause retinal injuries, whilst Ho:YAG may cause corneal injuries.

| VIVA | You may be asked in the FRCS (Urol) how you would make your theatre LASER safe – I suggest covering the following points in your answer:

- LASER alert signs outside theatre doors should be switched on
- Theatre doors should be locked when LASER is in use
- Windows should be blacked out to prevent any reflection
- Safety goggles on all theatre staff and the patient
- Clinicians utilising LASER should have up-to-date LASER safety training certificate
- Minimise number of staff entering/exiting theatre
- Machine should be on standby at all times when not in use.

THEATRE DESIGN, CLEANING AND EQUIPMENT

DEFINITIONS

Sterilisation is the complete destruction of living organisms (including spores and viruses).

Disinfection removes most viable organisms but not necessarily all viruses and spores:

- Most commonly using moist heat or liquid chemicals
- Moist heat is safe and leaves no toxic residues, temperature typically 73–90°C
- Chemical disinfectants are either alkylating or oxidising agents.

Cleaning physically removes contamination but does not necessarily destroy micro-organisms.

Decontamination is a combination of processes that include cleaning, disinfection and/or sterilisation to render a medical device reusable and minimise risk of transmission of infection.

Levels of Disinfection

Disinfection of equipment is divided into three classes according to the Spaulding classification:

- *Critical* – these penetrate tissue (require sterilisation before and after use)
- *Semi-critical* – contact mucous membranes (e.g. cystoscopes)
- *Non-critical* – only contact intact skin (e.g. blood-pressure cuff).

AUTOCLAVING

Autoclaving is a process that combines heat and pressure to sterilise instruments (by combining pressure with heat, the temperature of water may be raised above boiling points).

Typical adjustable variables of autoclave machines are pressure, temperature and time.

A typical autoclave cycle would include 134°C for 3 minutes or 121°C for 15–30 minutes.

Flexible scopes cannot withstand the conditions of autoclaving (rigid scopes can), and they require high-level disinfection (soak time ≤ 30 minutes).

THEATRE DESIGN

A key principle in theatre design is the flow concept of a patient moving from outer "dirty" zone to clean zone between reception and theatre.

All used instruments and the patient should be moved back into the outer zone as soon as possible.

Prior to surgery, the patient should be pre-assessed early if possible and the presence of infections (e.g. MRSA, COVID-19) should be treated before their surgery.

Patient should have showered and any hair local to incision removed if it interferes with operation.

Operative site should have gross contamination before antiseptic skin preparation, and the antiseptic agent should be applied in concentric circles out towards the periphery.

Examples of skin prep agents include povidone-iodine (Betadine®) and chlorhexidine.

Ventilation

Theatre ventilation is provided by vertical or horizontal laminar air flow with positive-pressure air moving from clean to dirty environments.

Air goes through HEPA filters which remove particles > 0.3mm in diameter with an efficiency of 99.9%.

20–40 air changes/hour are normal but can be increased to 400 by a laminar flow hood.

An optimum temperature of 20–22°C and humidity of 50–55% should be set.

Warming blankets, bear-hugger, heating of IV and irrigation fluids are ways of maintaining patient's core temperature intra-operatively.

Air temperature in aseptic zone should be 1°C lower than clean zone to facilitate air movement.

THEATRE SAFETY

WHO Checklist

The WHO five steps to safe surgery include: [16]

(1) Team brief   (2) Sign in   (3) Time out   (4) Sign out   (5) Debrief.

List Planning

VIVA   You may be asked in the FRCS (Urol) to prioritise the order of a theatre list based on a list of different patients' needs and characteristics. As a guide you should consider the following:

- First: critically ill/sick patients
- Start of list: paediatric, pregnant, diabetic patients and/or those with latex allergy
- End of list: infected cases.

MRSA-positive patients where possible should be deferred, treated and relisted. If this is not possible then they should be placed last on the list.

Latex Allergy

For patients with latex allergy, all staff must wear latex-free gloves.

The anaesthetic tubing must be latex-free and cleaned as gas can carry particles – therefore place the patient first on the list or allow time after the preceding case to clean the tubing.

SUTURES

There are many variables when considering suture materials, including:

- Absorbable vs. non-absorbable
- Mono- vs. poly-filaments (mono- has less tissue trauma but less memory)
- Synthetic vs. natural.

Choice will depend on the type of tissues being approximated and surgical objective.

In closing abdominal wounds, a 4:1 ratio of suture to wound length is recommended.

In urological surgery there is a risk of non-absorbable clips/sutures/staples coming into contact with urine and becoming a nidus for infection or stone formation.

Table 3 – Different types of sutures and their properties [17]

Generic Name	Trade Name	Characteristic	Absorption Time	Use
Polyglactin	Vicryl (coated)	Synthetic, braided, absorbable	50–70 days	Tissue closure
Polyglactin	Vicryl rapide	Synthetic, braided, absorbable	40 days	Circumcision
Polydioxanone	PDS	Synthetic, monofilament, absorbable	180–210 days	Abdominal wound closure
Poliglecaprone	Monocryl	Synthetic, monofilament, absorbable	90–120 days	Tissue closure
Silk	Mersilk	Natural, braided, non-absorbable	N/A	Tissue closure
Polypropylene	Prolene	Synthetic, monofilament, non-absorbable	N/A	Vascular anastomoses

ENERGY IN SURGERY

Diathermy is the passage of high-frequency alternating current through body tissue, and where resistance/impedance occurs, heat is produced ≤ 1,000°C to cut/coagulate tissues.

Standard electrical current in UK alternates at around 50Hz.

At this frequency, current would be transmitted through body tissue but would result in excessive neuromuscular stimulation causing harmful electrocution.

Nerve/muscle stimulation ceases at 100 kHz, so diathermy is safe above this frequency.

Usual diathermy frequency is 400KHz–2.5MHz.

Tissue effects of diathermy:

- > 45°C causes protein denaturation
- > 90°C causes desiccation (slow) and vaporisation (fast)
- > 200°C all tissues reduced to carbon.

MONOPOLAR DIATHERMY

Monopolar diathermy involves the delivery of high-frequency current from a diathermy generator to the active electrode (e.g. forceps, resectoscope loop/ball).

Active electrode has small surface area (i.e. high current density) yielding heat at point of tissue contact.

Current spreads from this point throughout the body, returning to the generator via the patient electrode (earth) plate, which in practice is the diathermy pad placed on the patient.

This diathermy pad has a large surface area (current density is low, therefore minimal heat generated).

The pad should be placed on area of skin which is dry and hair-free to ensure contact is optimised.

BIPOLAR DIATHERMY

In bipolar diathermy the current passes down one limb of the forceps (active electrode) and back to the generator via the other limb (patient electrode plate).

There is no need for a patient pad to be placed when using bipolar diathermy.

Principle advantage is that current does not pass through body parts which are not being treated.

This allows greater precision as to which tissue is being coagulated (i.e. reduced thermal spread).

Bipolar should only be used for end-tissue procedures (e.g. penis) – with monopolar there would be risk that all current passes via common penile artery, eliminating sole blood supply to the penis.

Safety

Although bipolar is inherently safer than monopolar, both come with potential risks:

- Burns and explosions (e.g. if inflammable anaesthetic agents are used)
- Electrocution or nerve injury/stimulation (e.g. obturator kick)
- End artery and tissue necrosis
- Pacemakers/cardiac device disruption.

Risk of burns can be reduced by ensuring adequate patient plate placement, avoiding patient contact with metal objects (e.g. drip stand) and inflammable liquids (e.g. alcohol-containing skin prep).

Pacemakers and Diathermy

Surgery on a patient with a cardiac device/pacemaker should be approached with caution.

If proceeding with surgery is imperative, you must ensure surgical preparation involves:

- Full knowledge of device details (i.e. type, indication, insertion date) and last check date
- Review of cardiologist/cardiac physiology department letters
- Consider whether bipolar diathermy can be used alone.

ICDs should be switched to "monitoring only" to avoid inadvertent activation (and switched back to normal function after surgery).

The following strategies can be used to increase safety in cardiac device settings:

- Ensure patient diathermy plate is placed such that current does not flow through device
- Ensure optimal contact of diathermy plate
- Avoid grounding via ECG leads
- Use short bursts of diathermy only.

Cutting vs. Coagulation

As the waveforms of the current change so do the corresponding tissue effects:

- *Cut* waveform is high current and low voltage, producing heat very rapidly (> 200°C)

- *Coag* is a low intermittent waveform producing less heat so that a coagulum forms (> 45°C).

Blend settings exist, which are a combination of cut + coag.

Table 4 – Differences between cutting and coagulation diathermy [15]

Cutting	Coagulation
Continuous output (100% on)	Pulsed output (intermittent wave) (6% on)
Low voltage	High voltage
Intense heat (≤ 1,000°), more vaporisation	Less heat, more charring
Power 125–250W	Power 10–75W

Harmonic™ Scalpel

The Harmonic™ Scalpel uses ultrasonic energy rather than electrical current such as in diathermy.

Piezoelectric crystal for US generation is situated in the handpiece.

US controls bleeding at lower temperature (< 100°C) by instrument blade vibrating at ≥ 50KHz, compressing vessel walls followed by sealing with coagulation of a protein coagulum.

Has an active blade (lower blade and often curved) and a clamping upper blade.

Minimises smoke generation, tissue carbonisation and reduces risk of damage to collateral structures.

Ligasure

Ligasure is an electrothermal bipolar device which uses a combination of pressure compression and continuous bipolar energy to create vessel fusion.

Radio-frequency melts collagen and elastin in vessel walls and reforms it into a permanent seal.

Feedback system automatically discontinues energy delivery when the seal cycle is complete, preventing sticking or charring.

LAPAROSCOPY

Urological procedures continue to rely on laparoscopy, with operations performed both exclusively laparoscopically or in conjunction with robotic-assisted techniques.

Laparoscopic ports inserted preferably via Hasson/open cut-down technique and can be:

- Reusable or single use
- Sharp or blunt
- Available in varying sizes (5–15mm)
- Held in situ with inflatable balloon.

Complications of laparoscopic port insertion include:

- *Immediate*, such as bleeding and visceral injury
- *Late*, such as port-site hernia or bowel injury during port-site closure.

CO_2 is the gas of choice for insufflation during laparoscopy as it is non-combustible and physiological.

Prolonged CO_2 insufflation of the peritoneal cavity can cause:

- Decreased venous return
- Impaired intra-operative lung ventilation
- Gas embolus
- Vagal stimulation
- Abdominal/chest/shoulder discomfort in the post-operative patient.

STATISTICS

Sensitivity	- Proportion of patients who test positive among those who have the disease (rule in
	- No. of true positives / (no. true positives + no. false negatives)
Specificity	- Refers to test's ability to correctly reject healthy patients without a condition
	- Proportion of healthy patients known not to have disease, who test negative for it
	- No. of true negatives / (no. true negatives + no. false positives)
PPV	- Proportion with a positive test who actually have the disease
	- Positive predictive value = no. true positives / (no. true positives + no. false positives)
	- Depends on how common the disease is in the study population
NPV	- Proportion with a negative test who do not have the disease
	- NPV = no. true negatives / (no. true negatives + no. false negatives)
Type 1 error	- Inappropriate rejection of the null hypothesis
	- Indicates poor specificity (higher specificity yields lower Type-1 error rate)
Type 2 error	- Inappropriate acceptance of null hypothesis, often due to small numbers
	- Indicates poor sensitivity
Power	- Probability of achieving a non-significant result when the null hypothesis is true
	- Power ranges from 0 to 1 (as power increases, probability of making Type-2 error of incorrectly failing to the reject the null decreases)
Absolute risk	- Probability of an event in a particular group
	- (number of events in group) / (number of people in that group)

Relative risk - Ratio of probability of outcome in exposed group to probability outcome in unexposed group (incidence exposed / incidence unexposed)

- RR = 1 (exposure does not affect outcome)

- RR < 1 (risk of outcome is decreased by exposure)

- RR > 1 (risk of outcome is increased by exposure)

Odds ratio - Ratio of odds of A in presence of B and the odds of A without presence of B

- This statistic attempts to quantify the strength of association between A and B

NNT - Average number patients need to be treated to prevent one additional bad outcome

- NTT is the reverse of ARR

- NNT = 1/ARR

Levels of Evidence

1a   Meta-analysis of RCTs

1b   At least one good RCT

2a   Well-designed, controlled experimental study

2b   Well-designed quasi-experimental study

3   Well-designed non-experimental study e.g. case control series

4   Expert opinion

Grades of Recommendation

A -   Based on good-quality studies, including at least one RCT

B -   Based on well-controlled clinical studies but no RCTs

C -   Made in the absence of directly applicable studies of good quality

MISCELLANEOUS

BLOOD PRODUCTS AND FLUIDS

Packed Red Cells

A unit of packed red cells is 230–340mL and contains SAG-M (saline, adenine, glucose, mannitol) as the standard additive solution.

The SAG serves to maintain ATP levels whilst mannitol maintains membrane integrity.

Citrate is used to prevent blood from clotting (works by chelating calcium).

Donated blood is screened for HIV, hepatitis B/C, HIV.

Refrigerated shelf-life ~35 days.

Table 5 – Summary of ABO blood groups

Blood Group	Antigen on Cell	Antibodies in Plasma
O	None	Anti-A, anti-B
A	A	Anti-B
B	B	Anti-A
AB	AB	None

The complications of blood transfusion include:

- *Early:* allergic reaction, bruising, fever, acute haemolytic reaction, fluid overload
- *Late:* viral transmission.

Fresh Frozen Plasma

FFP is the fluid portion of a unit of whole blood.

Contains all endogenous coagulation factors except platelets (i.e. tissue factor pathway inhibitors, fibrinogen, protein-C, protein-S, anti-thrombin).

Major/persisting bleeding requiring blood transfusion means patient will become depleted of clotting factors which will need replacement.

FFP should be considered for use in the following circumstances:

- Clinically significant bleeding if patient has abnormal coagulation test results
- Prophylactic in coagulopathic patients about to undergo surgery with risk of significant bleeding
- Persisting bleeding in massive transfusion protocol.

FFP is stored in freezer (e.g. -40°C) and should be used as soon as possible after thawing.

Cryoprecipitate

Cryoprecipitate is a frozen blood product prepared from blood plasma.

It is rich in factors VIII and XIII, Von-Willebrand factor and fibrinogen.

Cryoprecipitate should be considered for use in the following circumstances:

- Clinically significant bleeding and fibrinogen level < 1.5g/L
- Prophylactic in patients with conditions such as haemophilia-A.

Stored in freezer (-25°C) for up to 36 months.

IRRIGATION FLUIDS

The body's osmolarity is ~280–295mOsm/L.

Normal saline (isotonic) – contains 154mmol/L of Na^+ and 154mmol/L of Cl^-.

1.5% glycine (hypotonic at 200mOsm/L) – is a non-ionic amino acid, used for monopolar surgery as it does not have free ions to carry charge from the electrode to the plate (saline has free ions).

RENAL IMPAIRMENT

Acute Kidney Injury

AKI is classified by measuring serum creatinine and determining the increase with respect to baseline:

Stage 1:	1.5–2x
Stage 2:	2–3x
Stage 3:	> 3x.

Chronic Kidney Disease

A patient can be diagnosed with CKD if they have abnormalities of kidney function or structure present for ≥ 3 months. [18]

CKD is classified based on the GFR (and level of proteinuria).

Table 6 – Classification of chronic kidney disease [19]

GFR (mL/min)	Stage of CKD
≥ 90	1
60–89	2
45–59	3a
30–44	3b
15–29	4
< 15	5

DIALYSIS

Recall the indications for emergency dialysis via mnemonic AEIOU – Acidosis, Electrolyte imbalance, Intoxicants, Overload, Uraemia.

Haemofiltration is more likely to be used in the emergency/ITU setting.

Haemofiltration

Haemofiltration uses a highly permeable membrane.

Slow rate of blood flow (i.e. pump is not required), but a continuous process ongoing 24 hours/day from an artery and fed back into a vein.

Relies on hydrostatic pressure gradient across the membrane, removing solutes by filtration.

It will produce an ultrafiltrate and the movement of solutes is by convection.

Membrane has comparatively larger pores, thus clearing more medium molecular weight solutes.

Haemodialysis

Blood is separated from dialysate by semi-permeable membrane.

Fast flow rate is required by pump to process large volumes of blood, as an intermittent process (e.g. 4-hour sessions, 3x/week).

Solute clearance is achieved by diffusion (speed depends on flow rate, osmotic pull, molecular size).

Cleaned blood is returned to the body and heparin is used to prevent clotting.

Peritoneal Dialysis

Peritoneal dialysis requires a surgical insertion of a peritoneal dialysis catheter.

Patient can flush 2–3L of dialysis fluid into the abdomen, using peritoneum as the membrane through which solutes and fluid are exchanged with blood.

After 4–6 hours the waste fluid is removed.

This process can be done continuously in "chronic ambulatory peritoneal dialysis".

Sclerosing peritonitis is a specific complication of peritoneal dialysis and involves bowel obstruction due to a thick fibrin layer within the peritoneum. [20]

Complications of Dialysis

Related to dialysis line – bleeding, pain, infection, clot/blockage, bacteraemia, endocarditis.

Dis-equilibration syndrome – consequence of large-volume fluid shifts (e.g. hypotension, fatigue).

Long-term sequalae – amyloidosis, cardiovascular disease, increased risk of renal cancer.

Steal syndrome – ischaemia from reduced arterial flow distal to the fistula, causing hand pallor/necrosis/pain/reduced function, and may require ligation of the fistula. [21]

HAEMOSTATIC AGENTS

There are many haemostatic agents used in surgery which can be based on collagen, cellulose, gelatin or polysaccharide spheres.

Floseal® is a flowable white matrix that is packaged in a pre-filled syringe and works as follows:

- Gelatin granules swell to produce tamponade effect
- High concentration of human thrombin converts fibrinogen to fibrin to form clot.

Tachosil® – haemostatic agent in the form of a patch which is available in different sizes and works as follows:

- Coated with fibrinogen and thrombin to promote coagulation cascade
- Placed on area with bleeding and gentle compression applied using a wet gauze.

Surgicel® – a family of different products including powder, gauze haemostat and melting haemostat, which are all based on cellulose.

VIVA   There are many haemostatic agents on the market. For the purpose of the FRCS (Urol) viva it is important to familiarise yourself with at least a few, such as the examples I have listed above.

MINIMALLY INVASIVE BOO PROCEDURES

Rezum®

The Rezum® device consists of a portable generator and a single-use disposable delivery device.

Radio-frequency energy is produced by the generator and applied to a conductive coil in the delivery device, producing thermal energy in the form of water vapour.

The steam is delivered to the transition zone of the prostate via a needle (penetration depth 10mm) to ablate the tissue and trigger cell necrosis.

Irrigation fluid of choice is normal saline.

Rezum® is further covered in Chapter 8, "Andrology & BPH".

UroLift®

UroLift® can be performed under local or general anaesthesia with antibiotics at induction.

The UroLift® system is comprised of 2 single-use components – delivery device and implants (made of nitinol/stainless steel).

One end of the implant is anchored in the urethra and the other attached to the outer surface of the prostatic capsule – usually 4 are required.

Contraindications include – active UTI, visible haematuria, large median lobe, prostate > 100cc.

Patients are safe to have an MRI scan after UroLift®.

Migrated implants can lead to bladder stone formation.

UroLift® is further covered in Chapter 8, "Andrology & BPH".

Prostate Artery Embolisation

PAE usually uses the femoral artery as access to the prostatic arteries, which are embolised with polyvinyl alcohol (PVA).

PAE was approved by NICE in 2018. [22]

PAE is further covered in Chapter 8, "Andrology & BPH".

REFERENCES

1. Napier-Hemy R (2012). Principles of Measurement of Urinary Flow. In: Payne S, Eardley I, O'Flynn K, *Imaging and Technology in Urology*, Springer-Verlag, London.
2. Allisy-Roberts PJ (2005). Radiation quantities and units – understanding the sievert. *Journal of Radiological Protection*, *25*(1), 97.
3. Little MP, Wakeford R, Tawn EJ, et al. (2009). Risks associated with low doses and low dose rates of ionizing radiation: why linearity may be (almost) the best we can do. *Radiology*, *251*(1), 6–12.
4. American College of Radiology (2020). Manual on Contrast Media. Available at: https://www.acr.org/-/media/ACR/Files/Clinical-Resources/Contrast_Media.pdf [last accessed 13 June 2020].
5. Royal College of Radiology – Standards for intravascular contrast administration to adult patients, third edition. Available at: https://www.rcr.ac.uk/sites/default/files/Intravasc_contrast_web.pdf [last accessed 13 June 2020].
6. Grobner T, Prischl FC (2007). Gadolinium and nephrogenic systemic fibrosis. *Kidney International*, *72*(3), 260–264.
7. Cornford P, Tilki D, van den Bergh RCN, et al. (2024). Available at: https://d56bochluxqnz.cloudfront.net/documents/full-guideline/EAU-EANM-ESTRO-ESUR-ISUP-SIOG-Guidelines-on-Prostate-Cancer-2024_2024-04-09-132035_ypmy_2024-04-16-122605_lqpk.pdf [last accessed 2 August 2024].
8. Ahmed HU, Zacharakis E, Dudderidge T, et al. (2009). High-intensity-focused ultrasound in the treatment of primary prostate cancer: the first UK series. *British Journal of Cancer*, *101*(1), 19–26.
9. Fritzberg AR, Abrams PG, Beaumier PL, et al. (1988). Specific and stable labeling of antibodies with technetium-99m with a diamide dithiolate chelating agent. *Proceedings of the National Academy of Sciences*, *85*(11), 4,025–4,029.
10. Jaffe RB, Middleton Jr AW (1980). Whitaker test: differentiation of obstructive from nonobstructive uropathy. *American Journal of Roentgenology*, *134*(1), 9–15.
11. Lupton EW, George NJ (2010). The Whitaker test: 35 years on. *BJU International*, *105*(1), 94–100.
12. Lawson R (2012). How to Do a Radioisotope Glomerular Filtration Rate Study. In: Payne S, Eardley I, O'Flynn K, *Imaging and Technology in Urology*, Springer-Verlag, London.

13. Bonkat G, Bartoletti R, Bruyere F, et al. (2024). EAU Guidelines: Urological Infections. Available at: https://d56bochluxqnz.cloudfront.net/documents/full-guideline/EAU-Guidelines-on-Urological-Infections-2024.pdf [last accessed 14 August 2024].
14. Niveditha S, Pramodhini S, Umadevi S, et al. (2012). The isolation and the biofilm formation of uropathogens in the patients with catheter associated urinary tract infections (UTIs). *Journal of Clinical and Diagnostic Research: JCDR*, *6*(9), 1,478.
15. Ellis G, Cohen D, Bycroft JA, et al. (2018). Urotechnology, Principles of Uroradiology and Miscellaneous. In: Arya M, Shergill IS, Fernando HS, et al., *Viva Practice for the FRCS (Urol) and Postgraduate Urology Examinations*, second edition, CRC Press, London.
16. Vickers R (2011). Five steps to safer surgery. *Annals of the Royal College of Surgeons of England*, *93*(7), 501–503.
17. Fawcett D (2012). Sutures and Clips. In: Payne S, Eardley I, O'Flynn K, *Imaging and Technology in Urology*, Springer-Verlag, London.
18. The Renal Association – CKD stages. Available at: https://renal.org/information-resources/the-uk-eckd-guide/ckd-stages/ [last accessed 14 June 2020].
19. National Kidney Foundation – How to Classify CKD. Available at: https://www.kidney.org/how-to-classify-ckd [last accessed 2 August 2024].
20. Rigby RJ, Hawley CM (1998). Sclerosing peritonitis: the experience in Australia. *Nephrology Dialysis Transplantation*, *13*(1), 154–159.
21. Wixon CL, Hughes JD, Mills JL (2000). Understanding strategies for the treatment of ischemic steal syndrome after hemodialysis access. *Journal of the American College of Surgeons*, *191*(3), 301–310.
22. NICE Guidelines (2018). Prostate artery embolization for lower urinary tract symptoms caused by benign prostatic hyperplasia. Available at: https://www.nice.org.uk/guidance/ipg611/chapter/1-Recommendations [last accessed 14 August 2024].

UROLOGICAL IMAGING & PRINCIPLES OF UROLOGICAL TECHNOLOGY MCQS

1. What is the standard size of a microbubble used in contrast-enhanced US?

    A) 2–10μ
    B) 12–20μ
    C) 22–30μ
    D) 32–40μ
    E) 42–50μ

2. What is the correct approximate US frequencies used to visualise the prostate (trans-rectally), testes and abdominal organs?

    A) Prostate 3.5MHz, testes 3.5MHz, abdominal 12MHz
    B) Prostate 7.5MHz, testes 12MHz, abdominal 3.5MHz
    C) Prostate 12MHz, testes 7.5MHz, abdominal 3.5MHz
    D) Prostate 3.5MHz, testes 7.5MHz, abdominal 12MHz
    E) Prostate 7.5MHz, testes 7.5MHz, abdominal 3.5MHz

3. What is the half-life of technetium-99m?

    A) 3 hours
    B) 6 hours
    C) 9 hours
    D) 12 hours
    E) 15 hours

4. Which radionuclide decays to produce 99mTc?

    A) ^{99}Rh
    B) ^{99}Sn
    C) ^{99}Te
    D) ^{99}Mo
    E) ^{99}Ru

5. *Which of the following statements regarding MAG3 is correct?*

   A) 90% of MAG3 is extracted by proximal tubules, 10% is filtered by glomerulus
   B) 10% of MAG3 is extracted by proximal tubules, 90% is filtered by glomerulus
   C) 75% of MAG3 is extracted by proximal tubules, 25% is filtered by glomerulus
   D) 25% of MAG3 is extracted by proximal tubules, 75% is filtered by glomerulus
   E) None of the above

6. *What does EDTA stand for in the radioisotope assessment of GFR?*

   A) Eriochromodiaminotetrachloric acid
   B) Edetatedinitrilotetrasodium acid
   C) Ethaminodicarboxytetraphosphate acid
   D) Edoxydiphosphotetracyclinic acid
   E) Ethylenediaminetetraacetic acid

7. *Which bisphosphonate is radiolabelled with 99mTc to perform nuclear medicine bone scan?*

   A) KDP
   B) LNP
   C) MDP
   D) NDP
   E) ODP

8. *Which metal is more commonly used to coat ureteric stents in order to make them radio-opaque?*

   A) Cobalt
   B) Vanadium
   C) Bismuth
   D) Manganese
   E) Terbium

9. *What colour ring does a 12F urinary catheter have?*

   A) Red
   B) Orange
   C) Green
   D) White
   E) Blue

10. *What is the correct wavelength for a Thulium LASER fibre?*

   A) 1,000nm
   B) 1,500nm
   C) 2,000nm
   D) 2,500nm
   E) 3,000nm

11. *What is the correct wavelength for a Neodymium LASER fibre?*

   A) 256nm
   B) 512nm
   C) 1,064nm
   D) 2,140nm
   E) 2,512nm

12. *Which of the following would be the most acceptable set of parameters to autoclave a medical device to achieve sterilisation?*

   A) 121°C for 3 minutes
   B) 134°C for 3 minutes
   C) 147°C for 3 minutes
   D) 160°C for 3 minutes
   E) 173°C for 3 minutes

13. *Which of the following sutures is not absorbable?*

   A) Polyglyconate
   B) Polyglactin
   C) Poliglecaprone
   D) Polydioxanone
   E) Polypropylene

14. *How long approximately does it take coated vicryl to be reabsorbed?*

   A) 15 days
   B) 25 days
   C) 35 days
   D) 50 days
   E) 65 days

15. *What is the correct frequency used in surgical diathermy?*

   A) 20Hz
   B) 200Hz
   C) 2KHz
   D) 20KHz
   E) 2MHz

16. *At what approximate frequency does the Harmonic Scalpel vibrate?*

    A) 50KHz
    B) 65KHz
    C) 80KHz
    D) 95KHz
    E) 110KHz

17. *What is added into a bag of red blood cells to prevent this from clotting prior to being used for blood transfusion?*

    A) Heparin
    B) Coumarin
    C) Anti-thrombin II
    D) Citrate
    E) Protein-C

18. *What is the standard additive solution used in blood banking in the UK for packed red blood cell bag storage?*

    A) SAG-M
    B) TAG-N
    C) CAG-B
    D) DAG-R
    E) MAG-C

19. *Which of the following does FFP not contain?*

    A) Fibrinogen
    B) Albumin
    C) Protein-A
    D) Protein-C
    E) Protein-S

20. *Which clotting factors are found in cryoprecipitate?*

    A) VII and XII
    B) VIII and XIII
    C) VI and IX
    D) V and XI
    E) IX and X

BLADDER DYSFUNCTION & GYNAECOLOGICAL ASPECTS OF UROLOGY

URINARY TRACT INNERVATION

BLADDER MOTOR INNERVATION

The LUT is innervated by 3 sets of peripheral nerves:

- *Parasympathetic* pelvic nerves (autonomic nervous system)
- *Sympathetic* lumbar nerves (autonomic nervous system)
- *Somatic* pudendal nerves (somatic nervous system).

These nerves contain both afferent (sensory) and efferent (motor) axons.

Parasympathetic

Pre-ganglionic fibres located in S2–4 spinal segments: [1]

- Synapse with post-ganglionic fibres within detrusor muscle
- Provide excitatory input to bladder smooth muscle to cause detrusor contraction (i.e. motor)
- Provide inhibitory input to bladder neck/urethra (causing relaxation).

Sacral micturition centre (parasympathetic) stimulates detrusor contraction.

Sympathetic

Sympathetic cell bodies are located in spinal segments T10–T12 and L1–L2.

Innervate trigone, blood vessels of bladder, smooth muscle of prostate.

Pre-ganglionic fibres synapse with post-ganglionic fibres in the hypogastric (or pelvic) plexus:

- Main function is inhibition of parasympathetic pathways (i.e. inhibiting contraction)
- Provides contraction of outflow tract (stimulates contraction of pre-prostatic sphincter).

Somatic

The somatic nerve to the pelvic-floor musculature and external urethral rhabdosphincter (skeletal muscle) originates from S2–4 and is conveyed via the pudendal nerve.

The cell bodies lie in a distinct motor nucleus at same spinal level, called *Onuf's nucleus*, in the ventral part of the anterior horn of the sacral spinal cord. [2]

Image 1 – Motor supply to the bladder

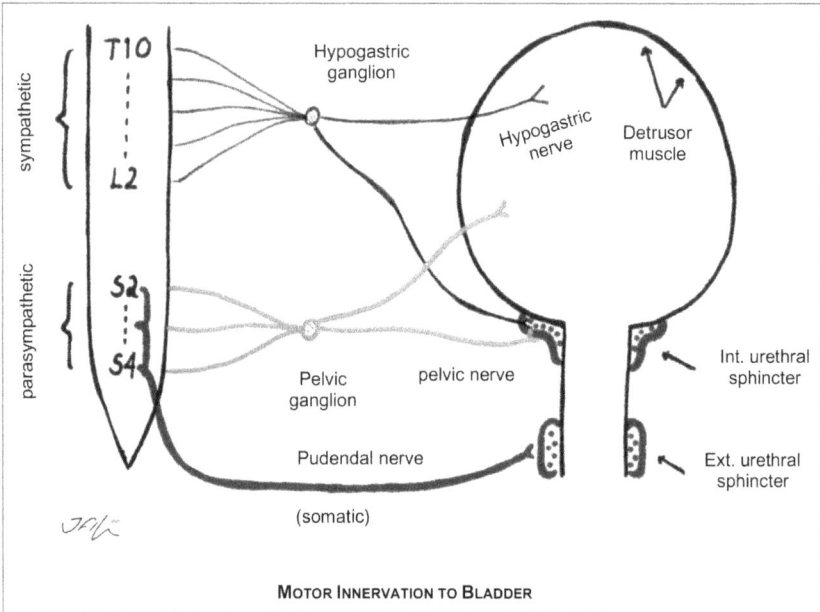

MOTOR INNERVATION TO BLADDER

BLADDER SENSORY INNERVATION

There are receptors throughout the bladder feeding afferent nerves, located in both detrusor muscle and sub-urothelial layer. [1]

Sensations of bladder fullness are conveyed to spinal cord in pelvic and hypogastric nerves.

Afferent nerves contain myelinated (Aδ) (respond to distension/contraction and filling information) and unmyelinated (C) fibres which respond to irritative stimuli and temperature.

Cell bodies located in dorsal root ganglia at S2–3 and T11–L2:

- Afferents enter spinal cord through dorsal horn
- Ascend to pontine micturition centre and cortex (via spinothalamic tracts).

Afferent fibres from trigone:

- Run in hypogastric nerve and ascend thoracolumbar cord to pons/cerebral cortex.

Afferent fibres from urethra

- Run in pudendal nerve and ascend thoracolumbar cord to pons/cerebral cortex.

The bulbocavernous (or bulbospongiosus) reflex checks the S2–4 arc: by squeezing the glans/clitoris or pulling on a urinary catheter, this should result in anal sphincter contraction.

URETHRAL SPHINCTER INNERVATION

The external urethral sphincter mechanism is distal to the apex of the prostate (between verumontanum and proximal bulbar urethra).

The external urethral sphincter has 3 components: [3]

1. *Extrinsic skeletal muscle*

   Outermost layer, pubo-urethral sling (part of levator ani), made of striated muscle, innervated by pudendal nerve (S2–4 somatic), augments urethral occlusion pressure

2. *Smooth muscle within urethral wall*

   Cholinergic innervation for tone, relaxed by nitric oxide

3. *Intrinsic striated muscle*

   U-shaped skeletal muscle within the wall of the urethra (rhabdosphincter) – absent posteriorly, produces occlusion by kinking rather than circumferential compression.

Pre-ganglionic somatic nerve fibres derived from S2–4 (Onuf's nucleus):

- Travel to rhabdosphincter via perineal branch of pudendal nerve for motor input
- Active nerves contract sphincter/inhibit micturition.

There is also input from pelvic plexus branches (i.e. not solely dependent on pelvic nerve).

MICTURITION CYCLE

FILLING PHASE

~98% of the micturition cycle is spent in the *filling* (storage) phase.

During bladder filling the intra-vesical pressure remains low – upper tracts may be in jeopardy once bladder pressures > 40cm H_2O.

Low pressure is maintained by bladder compliance ($\delta V/\delta P$) – mediated by its vesico-elastic properties.

These properties include its composition of elastin and collagen fibres, as well as the ability of detrusor smooth muscle cells to increase in length without significant increase in tension.

However, chronic obstruction/distension/raised pressure will lead to fibrotic changes and stiffening.

As bladder fills, afferent activity from stretch receptors passes to pons and cerebral cortex.

In the filling phase, when voiding is voluntarily inhibited: [3]

- Increased activity within external urethral sphincter
- Central inhibition to decrease parasympathetic activity to detrusor
- Gating mechanism within parasympathetic ganglia, whereby pre-ganglionic fibres inhibit afferent fibre activity via interneurons.

Guarding reflex is gradual increase in striated sphincter activity by increased pudendal nerve activity during normal filling, to match the rising urethral pressure. [4]

VOIDING PHASE

Micturition should be initiated when socially appropriate or convenient to the patient.

Stretch receptors in bladder sense increasing tension, which is relayed via afferent neurons to the dorsal horn of sacral cord and conveyed to periaqueductal grey matter.

The periaqueductal grey (along with input from other brain areas) feeds pontine micturition centre to determine whether it is appropriate to void.

If micturition is appropriate, it is co-ordinated by Barrington's nucleus (pontine micturition centre):

- EUS relaxation by somatic nerve inhibition in Onuf's nucleus
- Followed by detrusor muscle contraction (S2–4 parasympathetic).

In supra-sacral SCI the patient thus risks developing DetSD.

UROLOGICAL CHARACTERISTICS OF NEUROLOGICAL INJURIES

Many neurological conditions are associated with an abnormal bladder and sphincter function, and their symptomatology is defined as *neuropathic*.

The bladder and/or sphincter may as a result each be over- or underactive.

In healthy patients, the bladder and sphincter collaborate via a reciprocal relationship:

- During filling phase, the sphincter pressure is high and detrusor muscle is inactive
- During voiding phase, the sphincter relaxes and then detrusor muscle contracts.

Upper-tract jeopardy arises when there is uncoordinated detrusor muscle contraction working against a contracted sphincter, creating a high-pressure system.

In situations of *high-pressure bladder and high-pressure sphincter:* [5]

- Overactive bladder in the neuropathic patient is defined as *detrusor hyperreflexia*
- At times high bladder pressure overcomes sphincter pressure and patient leaks urine; however, the kidneys suffer back pressure, become hydronephrotic and eventually fail
- When sphincter pressure > bladder pressure, emptying is ineffective, leading to rUTI/retention
- An overactive sphincter generates high pressure during filling and voiding, which is termed DetSD.

In situations of *low-pressure bladder and high-pressure sphincter:* [5]

- An underactive bladder in the neuropathic patient is defined as *detrusor areflexia* – the bladder may simply fill up and not empty at all.

In situations of *high-pressure bladder and low-pressure sphincter:* [5]

- Bladder only able to hold small volumes of urine before leaking, resulting in incontinence.

In situations of *low-pressure bladder and low-pressure sphincter:* [5]

- Detrusor areflexia may make patient dry most of the time
- Incontinence may occur during raised abdominal pressure (as the sphincter is incompetent), for example during patient transfer from wheelchair.

Suprapontine Lesions

Examples of suprapontine lesions include CVA and Parkinson's disease.

Micturition reflexes are intact but leakage may occur at inappropriate times due to DO; however, pattern is normal and bladder pressures are safe.

Patient will suffer predominantly storage symptoms and UDS may show DO.

Supra-sacral Spinal Cord Injuries

SCI occurring between pons and L5 (i.e. between pontine micturition centre and sacral micturition centre) are considered supra-sacral lesions.

These patients experience both storage and voiding symptoms, and feature neurogenic DO and DetSD on UDS with poorly compliant bladders, which may result in unsafe high-pressure systems.

In lesions occurring above T6, patients may suffer the emergency condition *autonomic dysreflexia*.

Cauda Equina / Conus (S1–5) / Peripheral Nerve Lesions

Sacral/infrasacral cord injuries yield a lower motor neurone type of neurological pattern.

Characterised by areflexic bladder with urethral sphincter weakness (stress incontinence), the pressure is usually low, which is safer; however, the patient is likely to suffer with chronic retention.

Other Neurological Conditions

Multiple sclerosis – most common issue is NDO +/- DetSD, causing urgency/ frequency symptoms.

Parkinson's disease – most common issue is NDO; patients do not tend to have DetSD and therefore void unobstructed (unless they have BOO) [6] but tend to have poorer outcome after TURP.

Multiple system atrophy (formerly Shy–Drager syndrome) – this is a cause of Parkinsonism characterised by postural hypotension, the loss of pons cells causes detrusor hyperreflexia, the loss of Onuf's nucleus neurons denervates sphincter causing urinary incontinence. [7]

Spina bifida – results from failure of neural tube to close correctly; patients have combination of loss of compliance, DetSD and NDO; the mainstay of management is achieving low-pressure system to protect kidney function, achieve continence and QOL improvement.

AUTONOMIC DYSREFLEXIA

Autonomic dysreflexia is a potentially life-threatening medical emergency occurring only in SCI patients.

It may occur if SCI is above T6 (the sympathetic outflow) and is thus more common in cervical lesions.

Autonomic dysreflexia is a sudden and exaggerated autonomic (primarily sympathetic) response to a peripheral stimulus, which tend to be noxious and below the level of the SCI. [1]

Common stimuli that may lead to AD include: [8]

- Bladder distension/irritation (most common – 75%)
- Bowel distension/faecal impaction (second most common – 15%)
- Iatrogenic urological interventions, UTI, urolithiasis
- Non-urological causes can range from ingrown toenail to lower-limb fractures.

Pathogenesis

Noxious stimulus leads to sympathetic discharge, leading to reflex arterial vasoconstriction and consequently systemic hypertension.

Carotid bodies detect this rise in blood pressure and try to compensate with vagal reflex discharges, which cause vasodilatation and bradycardia as homeostatic response.

This compensatory stimulus, however, cannot cross the level of the SCI injury.

Vasoconstriction and hypertension persist – below the level of injury the patient is pale and clammy, above the level of injury they are sweaty and flushed.

Diagnostic Evaluation

From the patient history the following should be elucidated:

- Full details of the patient's SCI including level of injury
- Any previous episodes of autonomic dysreflexia
- Enquire for any potential noxious stimuli.

Patient examination in the presence of chaperone should assess for:

- Significant rise in systolic and diastolic blood pressure
- Profuse sweating and flushing above the level of lesion, usually face/neck/shoulders
- Pale clammy skin below level of lesion
- Abdominal examination for palpable bladder/DRE for faecal impaction.

Perform urinalysis +/- send MSU for culture, undertake bladder scan.

Management

The main principles of the management involve the following: [9]

- Prompt recognition of the condition
- Identification of precipitating factor and reversing this (e.g. catheterise if in retention)
- Sit patient upright (induce orthostatic hypotension)
- Administer sublingual GTN + IV labetalol +/- immediate release nifedipine
- Place on cardiac monitoring and involve critical care outreach.

If untreated, the hypertension seen in autonomic dysreflexia may lead to CVA, MI, haemorrhage, convulsions and patient death.

OVERACTIVE BLADDER

DEFINITIONS

OAB syndrome is a symptom syndrome of:

- Urgency with (OAB-wet) or without (OAB-dry) urge incontinence
- Usually accompanied with urinary frequency and nocturia
- In the absence of UTI or other detectable disease.

Idiopathic DO is a UDS diagnosis, whereby detrusor contraction(s) have occurred during filling cystometry, which may be spontaneous or provoked.

Urinary incontinence is the involuntary leakage of urine.

Urge urinary incontinence is the involuntary leakage of urine preceded by urinary urgency.

Stress urinary incontinence is the involuntary leakage of urine on effort/exertion.

Mixed urinary incontinence is the involuntary leakage of urine associated with urgency and exertion/effort.

Overflow incontinence is the leakage of urine when bladder is abnormally distended with large PVR.

Urethral hypermobility is a condition of excessive movement and instability of the female urethra due to weakened urogenital diaphragm.

EPIDEMIOLOGY

Estimated that ≤ 12% of adults experience OAB symptoms.

Urinary incontinence is twice as common in females vs. males.

In women the most common form of incontinence is SUI.

RISK FACTORS

Risk factors predisposing to urinary incontinence include:

- Gender – females are at higher risk
- *Race* – Caucasians higher risk than Afro-Caribbeans
- Neurological – such as MS, CVA, Parkinson's disease
- Childbirth, vaginal (forceps) delivery, increasing parity, pregnancy

- Pelvic surgery/radiotherapy
- Diabetes and rUTI
- Smoking/chronic cough
- Obesity, poor mobility
- Old age, cognitive decline, oestrogen deficiency.

DIAGNOSTIC EVALUATION

PATIENT HISTORY

A thorough patient history is the first step in the assessment of all patients with urinary incontinence.

The main aims of the history include:

- Trying to differentiate patient as having UUI, SUI or MUI
- Identifying (reversible) risk factors for urinary incontinence
- Enquiring regarding any red-flag symptoms.

The following points should further be elucidated:

- Duration and onset of symptoms
- Exacerbating factors
- Description of any episodes of urinary incontinence
- Number of pads required daily/impact on QOL
- Details on fluid intake
- Any concurrent bowel/sexual dysfunction.

A bladder diary should be completed for ≥ 3 days (EAU 2024).

Bladder diary records the type and volume of fluid intake, incontinence episode, number of used pads along with urinary frequency and voided volume.

FVC only records urine volume and frequency and incontinence episodes.

Nocturnal polyuria is diagnosed from a bladder diary by night-time urine volume (includes first morning void) and is diagnosed if ≥ 1/3 of the total urine volume over 24 hours is passed at night.

Validated patient-completed questionnaires are helpful, although there is no single questionnaire that fulfils all requirements for assessment of patients with incontinence.

VIVA If you are asked in your FRCS (Urol) viva to assess a patient with urinary incontinence, I recommend you state that you would see them in a dedicated functional urology clinic in the presence of a continence nurse specialist, asking patient to complete an ICIQ short-form questionnaire (Table 1) prior to entering the consultation room.

Table 1 – ICIQ-UI Short Form questionnaire for urinary incontinence [10]

1. Date of birth	
2. Gender	Female
	Male
3. How often do you leak urine?	0 – Never
	1 – once a week or less
	2 – 2–3x/week
	3 – about once a day
	4 – several times a day
	5 – all the time
4. How much urine do you usually leak?	0 – none
	2 – small amount
	4 – moderate amount
	6 – large amount
5. Overall, how much does leaking urine interfere with your everyday life?	0 1 2 3 4 5 6 7 8 9 10
	Not at all A great deal
ICIQ Score:	Sum of Q3, Q4, Q5 (0–21)
When does urine leak? (not included in score)	Never – urine does not leak
	Leaks before you can get to the toilet
	Leaks when you cough or sneeze
	Leaks when you are asleep
	Leaks when you are physically active/exercising
	Leaks when you have finished urinating and are dressed
	Leaks for no obvious reason
	Leaks all the time

PATIENT EXAMINATION

Both Sexes

A chaperone should be present for intimate examination in all patients.

Examine the abdomen for palpable bladder, scars and organomegaly.

Neurological examination should include assessment of gait, lower-limb function, perineal sensation and lower-spine visualisation/palpation.

Consider DRE to evaluate for constipation, palpable masses and anal tone assessment.

Women

Bimanual examination will reveal any pelvic masses.

Pelvic examination in the supine position should be undertaken to identify:

- Signs of vaginal atrophy/dryness associated with oestrogen deficiency
- Pelvic organ prolapse (consider POPQ – discussed in pelvic organ prolapse section)
- Digital assessment of strength of pelvic-floor muscle contraction (Oxford Grading System).

Pelvic examination in left lateral position with Sim's speculum should be undertaken to evaluate for cystocoele or rectocoele.

Cough stress test with sufficiently full bladder should identify presence of SUI.

The *Modified Oxford Scale* is a tool for evaluating pelvic-floor muscle strength via a 6-point scale (Table 2).

Table 2 – Modified Oxford Grading System for pelvic-floor muscle strength [11]

Score	Finding
0	No contraction
1	Flicker
2	Weak
3	Moderate
4	Good
5	Strong

INVESTIGATIONS

Initial Tests

Perform urinalysis +/- MSU culture if required.

If UTI present, treat with antibiotics and reassess incontinence following treatment.

Perform US KUB to assess PVR and hydronephrosis (EAU 2024). [12]

Consider flexible cystoscopy for persistent/severe symptoms, red-flag symptoms (visible haematuria and painful bladder), rUTI and voiding difficulties.

Pad Testing

The objective of a pad test is to try to quantify the volume of urine lost by weighing a perineal pad before and after provocation testing.

Pad test can be done as:

- Short term (1 hour): drink 500mL then proceed with exercise, ≤ 1.4g pad gain is acceptable
- Long term (24 hours): undergoing normal daily activity, ≤ 4g pad gain is acceptable.

NICE 2019 does not recommend pad testing as routine for women with urinary incontinence. [13]

Urodynamics

UDS is the mainstay investigation for assessing severe/refractory OAB symptoms.

UDS need not be performed to investigate uncomplicated OAB/UI/SUI.

Lifestyle implementations, bladder retraining, PFE and anticholinergics can be prescribed to treat presumed OAB without need for prior UDS.

NICE 2019 recommend that UDS should be undertaken if: [13]

- Symptoms of OAB leading to clinical suspicion of DO
- Symptoms suggestive of voiding dysfunction
- Previous surgery for SUI.

Consider UDS prior to any surgical intervention (recall that 16% of SUI also have DO on UDS).

Consider VUDS if presenting with neurological features, in children or previous failed surgery.

MANAGEMENT

CONSERVATIVE MEASURES

The following lifestyle measures should be proposed if applicable: [13]

- Optimisation of weight (weight loss improves UI in women) and regular exercise
- Treatment of constipation and chronic cough (along with smoking cessation advice)
- Avoidance of caffeinated or alcoholic drinks (may improve urge symptoms but not UUI).

Bladder Retraining

Bladder retraining is based on notion that central control can be relearned as in infancy.

It is done by setting target time for using toilet before which patient should not void, gradually increasing intervals of time, whilst maintaining normal fluid intake.

Bladder retraining is effective for improvement of urinary incontinence in women.

Effectiveness diminishes after the treatment has ceased.

NICE 2019 recommends bladder retraining be undertaken for ≥ 6 weeks as first line for UUI/MUI. [13]

Pelvic-floor Muscle Training

The aim of PFMT is to strengthen and rehabilitate the pelvic floor, increase tone and urethral resistance; however, it may also inhibit bladder contraction in OAB (i.e. not only benefit incontinence).

Regime involves long slow contractions and short sharp pull-ups at regular intervals.

NICE 2019 states PMFT should comprise ≥ 8 contractions performed 3x/day, for ≥ 3 months. [13]

PFMT may be undertaken electively in radical prostatectomy patients and pregnancy.

The addition of biofeedback to PFMT confers greater benefit in women.

Neurostimulation

NICE 2019 states that TENS should not be offered to treat OAB. [13]

EAU 2024 advises that electrical stimulation may improve symptoms of OAB; however, the type and mode of delivery are variable and poorly standardised. [12]

ANTICHOLINERGICS

Anticholinergic drugs are mainstay of treatment for UUI and OAB.

The agents differ in their pharmacological/kinetic profiles; however, there is limited evidence to suggest that one drug is superior to any other for QOL improvement. [14]

All anticholinergic drugs are superior to placebo in treating urinary incontinence; however, absolute size of effect is small.

The efficacy varies between 50% and 75% (they increase voided volume and decrease detrusor pressure).

Higher doses are more effective but with a higher risk of side-effects.

There is no demonstrable benefit in adding PFMT to anticholinergic drugs in treating UUI.

Adherence is low, most patients stop treatment within 3 months (due to inefficacy, side-effects or cost).

Commonest side-effect of anticholinergic drugs is dry mouth – others include constipation, blurred vision (accommodation paralysis), fatigue, cognitive dysfunction, prolonged QT interval.

Contraindications to anticholinergics use include:

- Myasthenia gravis
- Uncontrolled narrow-angle glaucoma
- Bladder outflow obstruction/high risk of urinary retention
- Active ulcerative colitis/toxic megacolon
- Bowel obstruction or intestinal atony.

Mechanism of Action

Acetylcholine acts on the muscarinic receptors on bladder smooth muscle which cause contractions.

Majority of muscarinic receptors in the detrusor muscle are M2 (however, M3 are the functionally important receptors).

Anticholinergic drugs are competitive muscarinic receptor antagonists and have high binding affinity mediating bladder contraction and reducing spontaneous detrusor activity during filling phase.

Selective anticholinergics block M1/2 receptors but not brain M1 receptors, thus are associated with a better side-effect profile.

Table 3 – Examples of anticholinergic drugs and their properties [1]

Trade/Generic Name	Dosage	Receptor Selectivity	Half-life
Detrusitol/ Tolterodine	2mg BD	Non-selective	2.4
Detrusitol XL/ Tolterodine	4mg OD	Non-selective	8.4
Regurin/Trospium chloride	20mg BD	Non-selective	20
Ditropan/ Oxybutynin chloride	2.5–5mg BD, QDS	Non-selective	2.3
Vesicare/ Solifenacin	5–10mg OD	Selective M2/M3	40–68

Association with Dementia

There is increasing concern that anticholinergic drug use has an association with developing cognitive impairment in the elderly.

This effect is not reversible, is cumulative in nature and increases with length of exposure, and is therefore termed the *anticholinergic burden*. [15] [16]

Oxybutynin in particular has been shown to worsen cognition in adults.

Small molecular size and high lipophilicity increase a drug's ability to cross the blood–brain barrier.

MIRABEGRON

Mirabegron is first clinically available β3-agonist drug.

β3-adrenoreceptors are the predominant β-receptors in detrusor smooth muscle cells and their stimulation induces detrusor relaxation.

Mirabegron is better than placebo and has similar efficacy to anticholinergic drugs.

Adverse events with mirabegron are similar to placebo.

NICE 2019 – mirabegron second line to anticholinergics (or first line if anticholinergics are contraindicated).

Blood pressure should be recorded prior to commencing mirabegron.

Contraindications to mirabegron use include:

- Severe uncontrolled hypertension (systolic BP ≥ 180mmHg, diastolic BP ≥ 110mmHg)
- Known hypersensitivity to agent.

Avoid usage in severe liver impairment and renal impairment (eGFR < 30mL/min/1.73m2).

Standard dose is 50mg OD (reduce to 25mg in mild liver impairment).

Side-effects of mirabegron use include:

- Arrhythmias
- UTI/cystitis
- Dyspepsia, skin reactions, joint swelling
- Hypertensive crisis (rare).

KEY PAPER | SYNERGY II Trial (2018) [17]

- Double-blind multi-centre trial of > 1,800 patients with OAB-wet.
- Randomised 4:1:1 to receive (mirabegron + solifenacin) vs. (solifenacin) vs. (mirabegron).
- Primary outcomes were safety + efficacy reducing number of micturitions and incontinence.
- Key finding was that combination therapy was safe and superior to either monotherapy.

If pharmacological therapy is ineffective, the patient should be referred for UDS.

Prior to offering invasive treatment for either OAB or SUI, the patient should be discussed in the appropriate local urogynaecology/pelvic-floor MDT.

MDT consists of sub-specialty interest urologist, urogynaecologist, physiotherapist, colorectal surgeon with special interest in functional bowel, continence nurse specialist. [13]

VAGINAL OESTROGEN TREATMENT

Topical vaginal oestrogen treatment is primarily used to treat OAB symptoms due to vaginal atrophy in post-menopausal women. [13]

Not associated with increased risks of VTE or breast cancer seen in systemic oestrogen therapy.

It improves urinary incontinence for post-menopausal women in the short term and should be offered.

Vaginal oestrogen should be prescribed on long-term basis – breast cancer is not an absolute contraindication; however, if history is positive the attending oncologist should be consulted first.

Ideal length of treatment remains unclear.

An example of a suitable vaginal oestrogen treatment regime includes:

- Consider first-choice Estriol 0.01% cream
- Apply once daily for 2–3 weeks
- Then reduced to twice weekly
- Discontinue every 2–3 months for 4 weeks to reassess need for further treatment.

BOTULINUM TOXIN

Botulinum toxin is a neurotoxin derived from Clostridium botulinum.

There are 7 serotypes all with similar pharmacological effects – types A and B are for clinical use (BOTOX is botulinum toxin A and 5x more potent than Dysport®).

BOTOX is indicated for treating NDO/IDO/DetSD, where these conditions have been proven by UDS and are refractory to conservative/medical therapy.

Benefit wears off over time; effect generally observed for 4–10 months (mean 6 months).

Botulinum A is much more effective in treating NDO compared to IDO.

Side-effects of intra-detrusor BOTOX include:

- Urinary retention (≤ 10% in IDO, higher in NDO ≤ 30%) i.e. patients must be taught ISC
- UTI, bladder pain, haematuria.

Contraindications to intra-detrusor BOTOX include:

Myasthenia gravis

- Concurrent use of aminoglycosides (e.g. gentamicin) which may augment effects
- Eaton–Lambert syndrome (auto-immune condition causing limb muscle weakness due to antibodies against pre-synaptic calcium channels at neuromuscular junction)
- Breast-feeding/pregnancy
- Bleeding disorders
- Inability to perform ISC.

Tolerance to the drug appears unchanged with repeated applications.

Regarding intra-detrusor BOTOX, NICE 2019 [13] recommends:

- Must be authorised by pelvic-floor MDT to treat OAB caused by DO proven on UDS where pharmacological therapy has failed
- Patient should be able to perform ISC or accept potential need for temporary indwelling catheter
- Use 100units of BOTOX-A as starting dose for OAB in women
- If symptom relief is inadequate, consider increasing dose to 200units.
- Do not offer botulinum toxin type B to women with OAB.

Mechanism of Action

Botulinum toxin A temporarily blocks pre-synaptic acetylcholine release at the neuromuscular junction of parasympathetic nerves supplying the detrusor muscle resulting in temporary paralysis.

It also prevents the exocytosis of acetylcholine by cleaving SNAP-25 off the SNARE proteins (a complex protein which when intact forms the core of neuro-exocytosis machinery).

The resulting chemical denervation is a reversible process.

Administration

Intra-detrusor BOTOX can be given via flexible or rigid cystoscope under local or GA.

The standard starting dose for IDO is 100units, for NDO it is higher at 200units.

Avoid injecting the trigone area.

There is no consensus regarding number and distribution of injection sites.

Do not give with gentamicin as can potentiate action of BOTOX and cause systemic effects.

KEY PAPER | DIGNITY Study [18]

- Randomised, double-blind placebo-controlled multi-centre study designed to evaluate the effects of onabotulinumtoxinA on urinary incontinence, UDS and QOL in NDO.
- MS (n = 154) and SCI (n = 121) randomised to placebo vs. 200units vs. 300units (1:1:1).
- Primary end-point – change from baseline in urinary incontinence episodes after 6 weeks.
- Secondary end-point – QOL score, UDS maximum cystometric capacity.
- Findings – significant reduction in urinary incontinence episodes and improved QOL in treatment groups; however, no significant difference noted between doses.

KEY PAPER | EMBARK Study [19]

- Randomised placebo-controlled trial studying OAB patients who failed anticholinergic treatment.
- > 500 patients who had ≥ 3 urinary incontinence episodes in 3 days were randomised to placebo vs. 100units onabotulinumtoxinA.
- Primary outcome – change in incontinence episodes, secondary end-point – QOL.
- Findings – treatment group superior in all OAB symptoms and QOL end-points.

POSTERIOR TIBIAL NERVE STIMULATION

PTNS device is connected near the ankle to stimulate the posterior tibial nerve, such that impulses travel to the sacral nerve plexus to modulate bladder function.

Given in out-patient clinic, 30-minute session per week, usually 12 sessions are offered.

NICE 2019 recommends that PTNS can be offered to women provided: [13]

- Authorised by the local pelvic-floor MDT
- Non-surgical/pharmacological management has not been successful
- Patient not accepting risks of BOTOX-A or SNM.

There is no current guidance on the use of PTNS in men.

SACRAL NEUROMODULATION

SNM is also known as *sacral nerve stimulation*.

SNM works by continuous mild electrical stimulation of afferents to bladder (mainly S3) modulating local neural reflexes and inhibiting bladder contraction.

SNM also affects higher brain centres involved in control of micturition.

Success rates ≤ 70%.

The side-effects of SNM insertion include:

- Local complications of bleeding and infection (if severe, may require removal)
- Pain at the site of implantation

- Discomfort in ankle or foot
- Adverse effect on bowel function
- Need for battery change.

NICE 2019 advises SNM can be offered to patients: [13]

- With OAB refractory to non-surgical management including medicines
- Provided this has been authorised by local pelvic-floor MDT
- BOTOX-A unsuccessful or patient unwilling to accept risks of BOTOX-A.

SNM Insertion

Can be performed under local or GA.

A two-stage technique is recommended to improve efficacy from 50% to 75%:

- Insert test wire into S3 foramina attached to temporary external pulse generator device
- Patient is discharged and asked to keep a bladder diary for ≥ 2 weeks
- If improvement of ≥ 50% is noted, proceed to insert a permanent electrode into S3 foramen with pulse generator in pouch superficial to posterior superior iliac crest.

Bilateral S3 nerve root stimulation for SNM has been proposed as an alternative for failed unilateral lead placement; however, the efficacy of this remains to be proven.

Assessing the patient with post-operative pain after insertion should include:

- Evaluating for any signs of infection
- Switching off SNM device (if pain settles this suggests it is due to electrical output)
- If no change by turning off, suggests cause is pocket related (e.g. size, erosion, seroma).

If symptoms return after an initial period of efficacy, check the battery and assess for lead migration by means of an XR.

A patient will not be able to have an MRI scan after they have an SNM inserted.

KEY PAPER | ROSETTA Trial [20]

- Multi-centre, open-label, randomised trial of 381 women with refractory UUI.
- Randomised 1:1 to (onabotulinumtoxinA) vs. (SNM).
- Primary outcome – change in mean daily UUI episodes.
- Key findings – both treatments helped reduce UUI episodes, BOTOX fared slightly better (reduction of 3.9 UUI episodes/day vs. 3.3); however, greater risk of retention and UTI.

CLAM AUGMENTATION CYSTOPLASTY

In clam augmentation cystoplasty the bladder is bi-valved (i.e. opened coronally) and the defect is patched with a detubularised segment of bowel.

Distal ileum is most common used (usually 25cm, starting 25cm proximal to the ileocaecal valve).

Any bowel segment can in theory be used if it has appropriate mesenteric length.

Cystoplasty will impair bladder contraction, lower detrusor pressures and increase bladder capacity.

The contraindications for performing clam augmentation cystoplasty include: [1]

- Severe inflammatory bowel disease
- Previous pelvic RTx
- Short bowel
- Inability to perform ISC
- Significant renal impairment (cannot compensate hyperchloraemic metabolic acidosis)
- Significant hepatic impairment.

The post-operative complications of clam augmentation cystoplasty include: [1]

- Pain/infection/bleeding
- Wound dehiscence/fistula
- MI/VTE/anaesthetic complications
- Small bowel obstruction/anastomotic leak
- Mortality $\leq 2.5\%$.

Biochemical Sequalae

Ammonium chloride (NH_4Cl) is absorbed by the clammed bowel segment -> $NH3 + HCl$

- And then HCl -> $H+ + Cl-$ (i.e. hyperchloraemic acidosis).

The acidosis is usually not clinically important (however, if significant then treat with bicarbonate).

This problem does not happen with ileal conduits, because urine passes through them and therefore does not have time to be absorbed, whilst a cystoplasty acts as a reservoir).

Long-term Sequalae

There are many potential long-term sequalae following clam augmentation cystoplasty:

- Need for CISC – increases over time
- Urolithiasis – more common in context of Mitrofanoff
- Mucus production – remains constant over time and can lead to rUTI, stones, blockages
- Bacteriuria – almost 100% of patients will have asymptomatic bacteriuria
- Deterioration of renal function
- Bladder perforation – high associated mortality due to frequent delay in diagnosis
- Risk of cancer – a longer-term risk, usually adenocarcinoma in region of the anastomosis
- Bowel changes – diarrhoea and low B12/folate (no terminal ileum absorption)
- Reduced growth potential – the H+ (from the acidosis) is buffered in exchange for Ca^{2+} causing bone demineralisation (osteopaenia).

STRESS INCONTINENCE

SUI is the involuntary leakage of urine on effort/exertion.

50% of all urinary incontinence in women is SUI.

UDS stress incontinence is defined as involuntary leakage of urine during increases in abdominal pressure in absence of detrusor contraction noted on UDS.

Intrinsic sphincter deficiency is the primary underlying cause for SUI in women (extrinsic urethral sphincter is not the primary mechanism for continence).

DIAGNOSTIC EVALUATION

PATIENT HISTORY

The patient should be seen in dedicated functional urology clinic with continence nurse specialist.

Consider prior completion of bladder diary over ≥ 3 days, a validated symptom questionnaire (e.g. ICIQ-SF – see "Overactive Bladder" section), urinalysis, PVR assessment.

A thorough history should be taken, as per OAB; however, regarding SUI in particular:

- Trying to distinguish between SUI, UUI or MUI
- Identifying SUI risk factors (obesity, chronic cough/constipation, multiple vaginal deliveries with instrumentation, previous pelvic surgery/radiotherapy, oestrogen withdrawal)
- Assessing for co-existing neurological conditions
- Enquiring about past urological history.

PATIENT EXAMINATION

All patient examinations should be performed in the presence of a chaperone.

Examination should be performed as per OAB; however, regarding SUI in particular:

- Supine pelvic, for oestrogen status, cough test, pelvic-floor tone assessment (Oxford grading)
- Left lateral position, for cystocoele and rectocele
- Evaluate PVR.

INVESTIGATIONS

Perform urinalysis +/- send MSU for culture if appropriate.

If UTI present, treat with antibiotics and reassess UI following successful treatment.

US KUB may be performed to assess for PVR, hydronephrosis or thickened bladder.

Consider flexible cystoscopy for persistent or severe symptoms, red-flag symptoms (VH and painful bladder), rUTI and voiding difficulties.

NICE 2019 does not recommend pad testing as part of routine assessment for women with UI. [13]

NICE 2019 does not recommend UDS be mandatory to investigate uncomplicated SUI. [13]

Lifestyle measures, bladder retraining/PFMT can be prescribed to treat SUI without prior UDS.

NICE 2019 suggests that UDS should be undertaken to investigate SUI if: [13]

- Urge-predominant MUI or type of urinary incontinence is not clear
- Symptoms suggestive of voiding dysfunction
- Previous surgery for SUI.

Consider UDS prior to any SUI surgical intervention (recall that 16% of SUI also have DO on UDS):

- If VLPP < 60cm H_2O, consider intrinsic sphincter deficiency
- If VLPP > 90cm H_2O, consider anatomical cause.

Blaivas and Olson classification is a tool to classify SUI based on VUDS, describing the position of the bladder neck and urethra, and is occasionally used. [21]

MANAGEMENT

Prior to offering invasive treatment for either OAB or SUI, the patient should be discussed in the appropriate local urogynaecology MDT.

Patient should be provided with *NICE patient decision aid on surgery for stress urinary incontinence.*

Surgical options include: bulking agents, autologous sling, colposuspension, AUS or diversion.

> **VIVA**   You should always state that you would provide the patient with the NICE patient decision aid on surgery for SUI in a FRCS (Urol) viva scenario about SUI. I recommend that you read and familiarise yourself with this 17-page document, which is freely available on the internet.

CONSERVATIVE MEASURES

Lifestyle advice is paramount and should be discussed:

- Weight loss, exercise, dietary advice
- Smoking cessation/treatment of chronic cough and constipation
- Fluid intake – avoid caffeinated drinks, moderate volumes.

PFMT should be undertaken by 8 contractions, 3x daily, for minimum 3 months.

The patient should be referred to the local community continence team for implementation and supervision of the advice above.

Vaginal oestrogen therapy can be offered to post-menopausal women with SUI.

DULOXETINE

Duloxetine is the only agent with published data available as medical therapy for SUI.

Duloxetine inhibits pre-synaptic reuptake of neurotransmitters (serotonin 5-HT and norepinephrine) at the spinal-cord level (Onuf's nucleus).

Mechanism of action is to increase activity of pudendal nerve and urethral muscle tone.

Prescribed as 20 or 40mg BD (PO).

Side-effects are common and account for the high discontinuation rates:

- Dry mouth, constipation, nausea
- Dizziness, insomnia and fatigue.

Duloxetine should not be offered as first-line treatment for SUI due to side-effect profile; consider as alternative option to SUI surgery if patient is unfit or unwilling (NICE) (EAU 2024).

BULKING AGENTS

The injection of bulking materials into bladder neck and peri-urethral muscles is a minimally invasive technique to increase outlet resistance.

Main indication is SUI in women due to intrinsic sphincter deficiency with normal detrusor function.

Other indications include patient preference, medically unfit for surgery, previous failed procedures and mild/moderate SUI.

Contraindicated if active UTI, concomitant DO and bladder neck stenosis.

The complications of injection of bulking agents include:

- Temporary urinary retention requiring ISC (10%)
- Failure to improve symptoms/need for further injections ($\leq$ 50%)
- UTI/VH.

Results tend to deteriorate with time and repeat treatments are often needed.

Bulking agents are less effective than surgery for treating SUI (however, lower complication rates) and should not be offered to those patients seeking permanent cure.

No bulking agent is known to be superior to any other; consider Macroplastique (silicone) as there is no significant risk of migration due to particle size.

Options for bulking agents include Bulkamid® and Macroplastique®.

VIVA You may be asked in your FRCS (Urol) viva how you would
perform bulking-agent injection to treat SUI. I recommend
watching an online video of the procedure, as many candidates
may not have seen this done before in clinical practice. I would
mention the following key points:

- WHO checklist complete, patient prepped + draped in lithotomy
position, under GA
- Induction antibiotic IV gentamicin administered
- Perform full diagnostic cystoscopy
- 2mg Bulkamid® given in 4 divided doses (12, 3, 6 and 9 o'clock) 1cm
distal to bladder neck.

KEY PAPER TVT vs. Bulkamid® – Freitas et al. in *Journal of Urology* (2020)
[22]

- 224 primary SUI women randomised 1:1 to (TVT) vs. (Bulkamid®).
- Primary outcome – patient satisfaction at 12 months (95% TVT vs. 60%
Bulkamid®); secondary outcome – cough test negative at 12 months
(95% TVT vs. 66% Bulkamid®).
- Key findings were Bulkamid® not as good as previously thought but
associated with lower complication rates.

MID-URETHRAL SLINGS

Mid-urethral slings are most frequently used surgical intervention for SUI in
Europe.

They work by impeding the movement of the posterior urethral wall.

Mid-urethral slings can be classified into:

- *Autologous:* rectus fascia, fascia lata
- *Synthetic:* prolene
- *Allograft*/cadaveric.

Synthetic slings can be placed via retropubic (TVT) or trans-obturator (TOT)
routes as day case.

Due to sustained concerns that have been raised and following the
Cumberlege Report in 2020, currently (as of 2024) mesh surgery for SUI
cannot be performed in the NHS.

Techniques of sling insertion included TVT and TOT.

The complications of TVT slings include:

- Bladder perforation
- Severe bleeding
- Injury to blood vessels/bowel/nerve
- Material related e.g. erosion/migration into urethra, bladder, rectum
- Voiding dysfunction including urinary retention, unresolved SUI.

TVT and TOT have equivalent patient-reported outcomes (cure rates).

Compared to TVT, the TOT procedure has:

- Lower risk of bladder perforation and voiding dysfunction
- Higher risk of vaginal injuries, groin/thigh pain and mesh erosion.

Mesh Complications

Since the Cumberlege Report, specialist mesh centres in the UK have been set up to provide comprehensive treatment for mesh complications.

Any patient with mesh complications should be referred to the appropriate regional mesh centre.

Addition of patient to pelvic-floor registry is encouraged.

Mesh eroded into vagina is termed *exposure*, whilst if into urinary tract it is called *extrusion*.

Autologous Slings

Most commonly a segment of rectus fascia measuring 10–20cm in length is harvested via Pfannensteil incision, non-absorbable long sutures placed on both ends.

The sling is placed under mid-urethra.

Sutures placed through endopelvic fascia up to remaining rectus tied using correct tension.

Autologous slings are more effective than colposuspension for improving SUI (EAU 2024).

Colposuspension

Retropubic suspension surgery used to treat female SUI mainly caused by urethral hypermobility.

The surgical principle is re-elevation of bladder neck into the abdominal pressure zone so there is equal transmission of pressure to bladder neck to close off the urethra.

The following patients may benefit from colposuspension:

- Young patient with SUI (due to current concerns regarding long-term use of mesh)
- SUI with significant urethral hypermobility.

Burch colposuspension is the most widely used procedure for this purpose.

Can be performed open/laparoscopic/robotic, with similar efficacy rates.

The complications after Burch colposuspension include:

- Immediate – retropubic space haemorrhage, bladder trauma
- Delayed – rectocoele ($\leq$ 20%), dyspareunia, voiding dysfunction and need for ISC, rUTI.

The alternative Marshall-Marchetti-Krantz procedure is not recommended by NICE.

KEY PAPER Burch Colposuspension vs. Fascial Sling, Albo et al. in *NEJM* (2007) [23]

- Multi-centre randomised clinical trial of 655 women with SUI.
- Randomised 1:1 to undergo (Burch) vs. (autologous fascial sling).
- Primary outcome was success across multiple urinary-incontinence measuring tools.
- Key finding was autologous sling was superior in treating SUI but had greater morbidity.

Artificial Urethral Sphincter

NICE 2019 recommends AUS be offered to treat SUI only after previous surgery has failed.

Can be inserted open/laparoscopic/robotic.

AUS cuff is placed around bladder neck, reservoir placed in space of Retzius and pump tunnelled in the labia majora.

High success rates but with the potential following risks:

- Urinary retention, voiding dysfunction, new OAB symptoms
- Urethral atrophy/extrusion, vaginal exposure
- Mechanical failure.

POST-PROSTATECTOMY INCONTINENCE

DIAGNOSTIC EVALUATION

History

The history for evaluating sphincter damage and symptoms should include:

- Causative procedure – RP (open vs. robotic vs. laparoscopic), TURP, pelvic RTx, pelvic fracture
- Details of cancer status e.g. PSA, margin status, planned adjuvant treatments
- Determining type of incontinence (SUI vs. UUI) and impact on QOL
- Presence of red-flag symptoms
- Overall fitness, hand function and cognitive status.

Patient should be encouraged to complete ICIQ-SF questionnaire (or equivalent) prior to clinic.

Patient should complete bladder diary.

Duration of symptoms following RP is important; most patients will have regained their continence within 12 months of surgery.

Examination

Record BMI.

Perform urinalysis +/- MSU for culture if appropriate – if positive, treat with antibiotics and reassess.

Examine abdomen (palpable bladder, scars), external genitalia (meatus, foreskin) and *cough stress test* whilst patient is standing.

Investigations

Request uroflowmetry with PVR.

Complete 24-hour pad weight test with following guide to categorisation of leakage severity:

- < 200mL/day (*mild*)
- 200–500mL/day (*moderate*)
- > 500mL/day (*severe*).

The key investigation is VUDS, which typically reveals stable compliant bladder with evidence of SUI; compliance, however, may be reduced if patient had previous RTx.

MANAGEMENT

Conservative options should be advised initially:

- Weight loss, exercise, diet, smoking cessation
- Supervised PFMT
- Bladder retraining and fluid advice (treats UUI component).

Penile clamp compressive devices can be used for pure sphincter urinary incontinence in frail patients.

Penile clamps have to be released frequently and should not be worn at night.

Duloxetine is option for men with SUI (EAU 2024) but counsel patient regarding side-effects.

Once sufficient time passed for natural continence recovery and conservative measures failed, post-prostatectomy incontinence men should be counselled regarding surgical treatment options.

Bulking agents have limited efficacy and are not recommended by EAU 2024.

Male Slings

The following male slings have been introduced to treat post-prostatectomy incontinence:

- *Non-adjustable* – positioned under urethra and fixed by a retropubic or trans-obturator approach, tension adjusted intra-operatively (weak recommendation by EAU 2024)
- *Adjustable* – sling tension can be changed post-operatively (supporting evidence is limited)
- Autologous (supporting evidence is limited).

No particular sling has demonstrated superiority over others

ARTIFICIAL URETHRAL SPHINCTER

AUS is the standard treatment for moderate-to-severe male SUI and can be used for all degrees of post-prostatectomy incontinence.

The AMS 800 is the device with the longest follow-up and greatest level of evidence.

The AUS is a closed pressurised system with 3 key components:

- Urethral cuff, placed around the bulbar urethra or bladder neck
- Activating control pump, placed in the scrotum
- Reservoir, placed extra-peritoneally in the abdomen (provides constant pressure to cuff).

The cuff provides a constant circumferential pressure to compress the urethra and is derived from the reservoir which is normally set at 61–70cm H_2O.

To void, the pump is squeezed which transfers fluid to reservoir balloon, deflating the cuff which then refills within 3 minutes (the time interval during which patient must void).

Efficacy is 75% completely dry and 90% socially continent, 60% have benefits for > 10 years.

The complications of AUS insertion include:

- Infection (most common pathogen is Staph. epidermidis)
- Cuff erosion, urethral atrophy (most common cause of surgical revision)
- Persistent leakage, mechanical failure.

Atrophy presents with gradual de-novo incontinence, mechanical failure with rapid onset incontinence.

Erosions/infections of AUS require device removal; do not reinsert for ≥ 3 months.

Always ensure the AUS is deactivated prior to any urethral instrumentation.

KEY PAPER | MASTER Trial (2021) [24]

- RCT, unblinded trial of 380 men with symptomatic UDS SUI.
- Randomised 1:1 to (trans-obturator sling) vs. (AUS) with outcomes at 12-months follow-up.
- Primary – patient-reported SUI; secondary – adverse events.
- Key findings were that SUI rates remained high although both treatments helped; no statistical difference in benefit between sling or AUS; however, AUS favoured in terms of complications.

URODYNAMICS

UDS (or VUDS) is the only method that can objectively assess LUT function.

In neuropathic patients UDS interpretation can be more challenging, and same-session repeat UDS are crucial as repeat measurements may yield different results.

In patients at risk of autonomic dysreflexia, monitor their blood pressure during UDS.

DEFINITIONS

The following are useful definitions when interpreting UDS:

Bladder compliance – relationship between change in bladder volume (ΔV) and change in detrusor pressure (ΔP_{det}), where compliance is ($\Delta V / \Delta P_{det}$).

Cystometric capacity (bladder volume) – urine volume at the end of the filling phase.

Detrusor overactivity – involuntary detrusor contractions during filling phase (diagnosis of DO can be made irrespective of the size of the contractions).

Neurogenic DO is DO in presence of an underlying neurological condition.

Terminal DO – single detrusor contraction at cystometric capacity which results in flooding.

Detrusor sphincter dyssynergia – detrusor contraction concurrent with involuntary contraction of urethral striated muscle which affects flow.

Abdominal leak-point pressure – intra-vesical pressure at which urine leakage occurs due to increased abdominal pressure in absence of detrusor contraction.

Detrusor leak-point pressure – the lower detrusor pressure at which urine leakage occurs.

Urethral pressure – the fluid pressure needed to just open a closed urethra.

Urethra pressure profile – a graph indicating intraluminal pressure along length of urethra.

INDICATIONS

There are many indications for performing UDS, including:

- Persistent LUTS after appropriate therapy (e.g. BOO surgery, medications)
- Previous failed incontinence surgery
- Mixed urinary symptoms +/- incontinence.

VUDS should be used in neuropathic patients, children and suspected SUI in post-prostatectomy incontinence, or in recurrent SUI after treatment.

In patients with new SCI, once the upper tracts are safe (e.g. SPC, LTC) they should be referred for UDS to provide baseline trace as they are at risk of neuropathic bladder changes in the future.

If patient has active UTI, this should be fully treated and UDS postponed until resolved.

Pause any medications prior to UDS that may interfere with trace reliability (e.g. anticholinergics).

TECHNIQUES

UDS should be performed in dedicated room with specialised equipment (VUDS requires fluoroscopy).

Perform urinalysis to exclude infection prior to commencing the study.

1. Uroflowmetry and PVR
   - Begin with flow-rate test to provide a first impression of voiding function. [1]

2. UDS Setup
   - Clean external urethral meatus, pass anaesthetic gel, insert dual-lumen 6–8F catheter into the bladder (to record intra-vesical pressure) and drain bladder (note the PVR).
   - Insert single-lumen catheter into rectum to record abdominal pressure.
   - Connect lines to urodynamic transducers and flush these with saline to remove any air bubbles.
   - Zero all lines to atmosphere, place transducers at level of pubic symphysis, make patient cough several times to ensure adequate subtraction (P_{det} < 6cm / H_2O at rest).
   - Detrusor pressure (P_{det}) = (intra-vesical pressure) – (abdominal pressure).

3. Filling Cystometry

    *   Only method for quantifying the patient's filling function – start with empty bladder.

    *   Fill slowly at physiological rate (20mL/s for neuropaths, 50mL/s for adults) using warm saline (or contrast medium in VUDS), cough every minute to review subtraction.

    *   Normal pressures at rest: P_{det} 0–6cm H_2O, Pves and Pabd 15–40cm H_2O.

Note the following findings on the filling phase:

*   Volume of first sensation, first urge and strong desire, *cystometric capacity*
*   Evidence of involuntary detrusor contractions (DO)
*   Evidence of slow rising intra-vesical pressure (poor compliance)
*   Incontinence and precipitating cause (SUI or UUI).

Filling phase historically described as having 4 distinct parts (see Image 2):

I. Initial fill (unfolding, viscoelastic)

II. Tonus phase (viscoelastic)

III. Limit of compliance (viscoelastic properties exhausted)

IV. Voiding (now considered to be in voiding phase).

Image 2 – Distinct parts of the filling phase on UDS

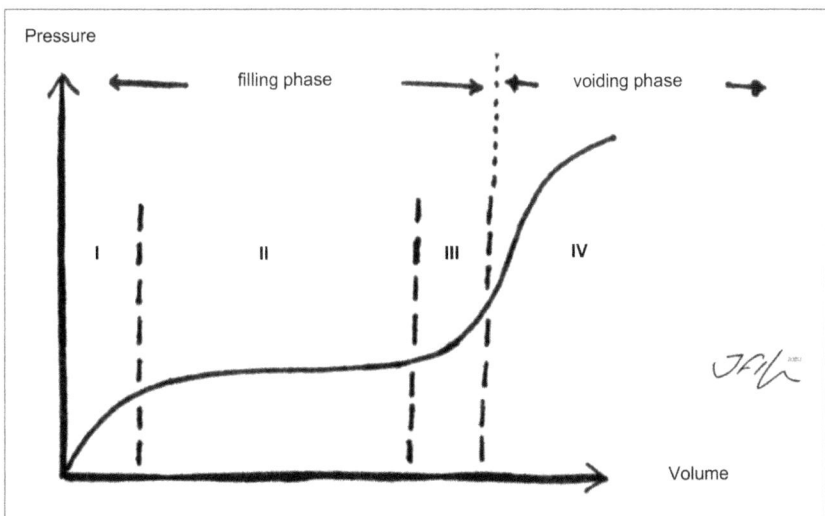

4. Voiding Cystometry

Pressure flow studies during the voiding phase reflect co-ordination between detrusor and urethra/pelvic floor – VUDS and filling phase should be interpreted alongside this.

Note the following findings on the voiding phase:

- P_{det} at Q_{max} and Q_{max} (determine BOO, bladder contractility index, detrusor failure)
- Voiding time and shape of curve
- Reciprocal relationship between voiding curve and P_{det} (DetSD).

VIVA   You may be asked in your FRCS (Urol) viva how you would perform a standard UDS test. I recommend covering the following key points:

- Ensure patient is suitably consented and changed into hospital gown, no infection present on urinalysis, any medications such as anticholinergics have been paused
- Urology nurse present
- Insert 6F dual-lumen catheter into urethra and rectum, document PVR
- Position taps to ensure pressure is zeroed to atmosphere
- Ensure adequate subtraction by asking patient to cough several times ($P_{det} < 6cm/H_2O$)
- Commence filling bladder at 50mL/min (20mL/min in neuropaths), check subtraction regularly, document any contractions, incontinence episodes or rise in pressure
- Enquire about patient desire to void (first and strong)
- Ask patient to void and determine flow shape, Q_{max} and P_{det} at Q_{max}.

Bladder contractility index = $P_{det}Q_{max} + 5Q_{max}$

BCI > 150 = strong contractility

BCI 100–150 = normal contractility

BCI < 100 = weak contractility

Bladder contractility nomogram – the patient can be plotted on the nomogram to determine whether their BCI is weak, normal or strong (see Figure 1). [25]

Figure 1 – Bladder contractility nomogram

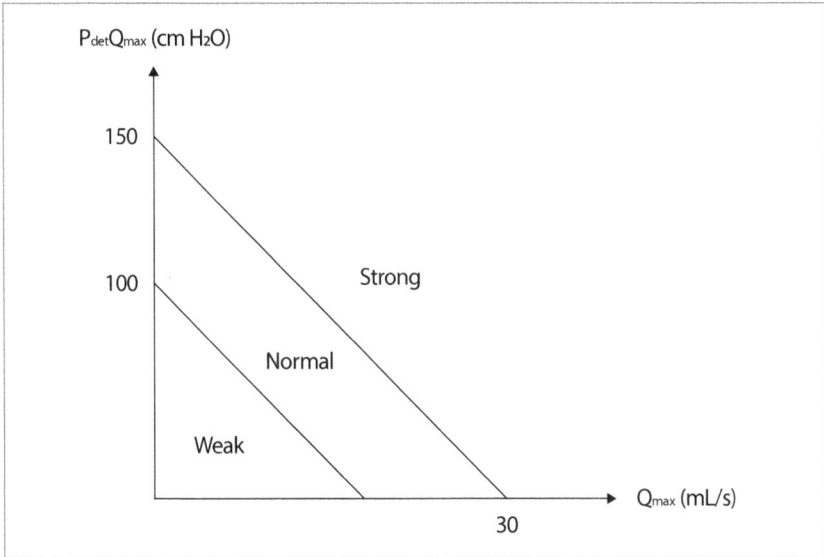

Bladder outlet obstruction index

(also Abrams–Griffiths number) = $(P_{det}Q_{max}) - (2Q_{max})$

BOOI > 40 = obstructed

BOOI 20–40 = equivocal

BOOI < 20 = non-obstructed

The ICS nomogram can be used to plot the measurements during UDS to determine whether the patient is obstructed, unobstructed or in the equivocal range.

Figure 2 – Bladder outflow obstruction nomogram

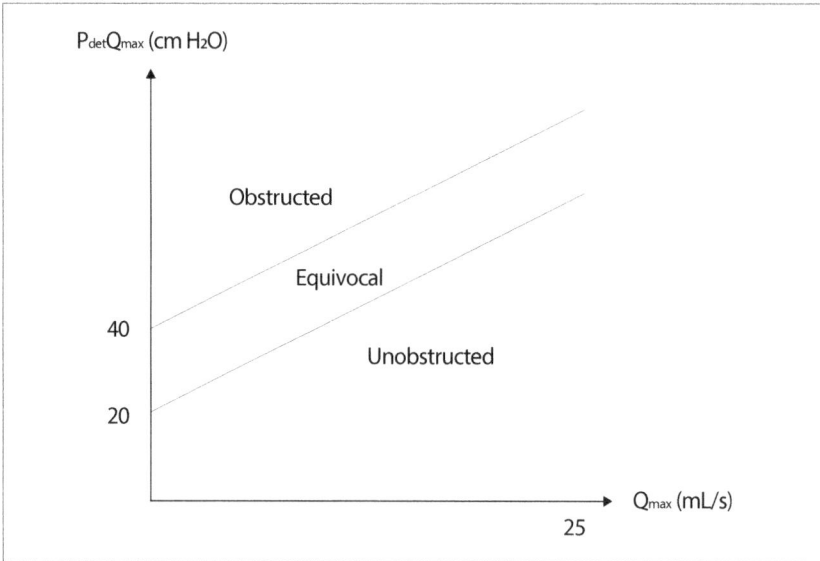

Loss of compliance defined as > 1cm H_2O rise in pressure per 40mL infused, standardised up to 400mL (i.e. no more than 10cm H_2O rise in pressure should be noted during filling phase).

The definitions and nomograms that are used to describe BOO in men do not apply to women.

In women there is no condition as common as BPH and therefore developing nomograms by similar methods is difficult.

Causes of obstruction in women vary from anatomical (e.g. POP) to functional (e.g. dysfunctional voiding) without one predominant diagnosis.

Leak-point Pressures

DLPP is the lowest detrusor pressure at which urine leakage occurs in the absence of either a detrusor contraction or increased abdominal pressure.

This term applies and should only be used in relation to neuropathic patients.

DLPP gives an indication of fixed outlet resistance.

DLPP > 40cm H_2O is associated with increased risk of upper-tract dilatation and deterioration.

ALPP (also *Valsalva leak-point pressure*) is the intra-vesical pressure at which leakage occurs because of increased abdominal pressure in absence of detrusor contraction.

ALPP is important in the investigation of SUI:

- ALPP < 60cm H_2O = significant intrinsic sphincter deficiency
- ALPP > 90cm H_2O = SUI likely due to urethral hypermobility
- ALPP > 150cm H_2O = urethra unlikely to be the cause of UI.

DETRUSOR SPHINCTER DYSSYNERGIA

DetSD is the involuntary contraction of the urethral and/or peri-urethral striated muscle simultaneously with detrusor muscle contractions.

DetSD is usually specific to supra-sacral neurological injuries or disorders.

Classic UDS trace in DetSD is *saw-tooth* appearance on P_{det} line which is sustained (e.g. > 5 minutes) with detrusor contractions having pressures 80–90cm H_2O.

Cystography at VUDS reveals a hold-up of contrast at the level of the external urethral sphincter.

DetSD jeopardises the upper tracts due to the high-pressure system it generates.

Treatment aims to reduce bladder pressures to safeguard the upper tracts and preserve renal function.

Management

Aim is to achieve low-pressure storage, achieve complete bladder emptying and promote continence.

Commence anticholinergic medication, teach patient ISC (or pass LTC) and monitor closely with repeat US at 3 months looking for upper-tract dilatation.

Repeat UDS after 3–6 months to ensure bladder pressures have come down.

Intra-detrusor BOTOX is an option; however, the patient would still need to perform ISC.

Augmentation cystoplasty +/- Mitrofanoff channel is an option; however, the patient would still need to perform ISC.

VUDS should be repeated 3–6 months after cystoplasty.

FEMALE URETHRAL DIVERTICULUM

A FUD is an epithelialised outpouching of the urethral mucosa with a single connection (ostium) entering the urethral lumen.

Most are asymptomatic or misdiagnosed, so the true incidence is unknown.

Multiple in 10% of cases.

Most common malignancy found in a FUD is adenocarcinoma.

AETIOLOGY

Believed to arise secondary to infection of peri-urethral glands, leading to local abscess formation and eventual rupture into the lumen.

Glands are located posterolateral to peri-urethral fascia (proximal 2/3) and drain into distal 1/3.

FUD is rarely congenital; however, common acquired causes include:

- Traumatic vaginal delivery
- Previous urethral/vaginal surgery
- Repeated urethral instrumentation
- Peri-urethral (Skene's) gland infection (e.g. N.gonorrhoeae, E.coli).

FUD can be single, saddle-shaped or even circumferential.

DIAGNOSTIC EVALUATION

Patient History

FUD presents with classic "3 'D's" (dyspareunia, dribble post-void, dysuria) only in 23% of cases.

- In clinical practice, patients present with a wide range of symptoms, therefore enquire regarding:
- Dysuria, dribble post-void, dyspareunia
- rUTI, visible haematuria, urgency
- Vaginal discharge
- Previous STI/instrumentation/local abscesses/previous urethro-vaginal surgery.

Patient Examination

Complete pelvic examination in the presence of female chaperone.

Evaluate for palpable lump in vagina which may discharge fluid (collect and send for culture).

Imaging

MRI is the gold-standard diagnostic imaging for diagnosing FUD. [1]

Sensitivity approaches 100% when used with endo-vaginal coil (i.e. not a surface coil technique) and allows localisation for surgical planning.

US (trans-vaginal/-rectal/-perineal) is less accurate than MRI but can be used as alternative.

MCUG has good sensitivity and allows concomitant assessment of any voiding dysfunction; however, the test exposes patient to radiation.

Cystoscopy

Use 0° or 30° scope and perform full diagnostic cystoscopy to check for other pathology.

Try to visualise the ostium of the diverticulum which may assist with surgical planning as this needs to be closed after diverticulectomy.

MANAGEMENT

Asymptomatic FUD does not require active intervention; however, patient should be suitably counselled as to common symptoms to look out for with underlying FUD.

Follow-up is advisable due to risk of malignant transformation.

Patients with LUTS, rUTI or pain symptoms may benefit from FUD surgery.

The principles of FUD repair (urethral diverticulectomy) include:

- Excision of diverticulum
- Closure of connection to the ostium
- Water-tight urethral closure with 4'0 vicryl +/- interpositioned Martius fat pad

- Preservation of continence (or alternatively insertion of sling device)
- Catheterisation for ≤ 14 days.

Complications from FUD repair include incontinence, urethra-vaginal fistula, urethral stricture, recurrent diverticulae and scarring leading to dyspareunia.

FEMALE URINARY TRACT FISTULAE

VESICOVAGINAL FISTULA

The most common type of urinary tract fistula is VVF.

VVF is an abnormal communication between the bladder and vagina.

Onset can be rapid (days/weeks) typically after surgical intervention or obstructed labour, or delayed (months/years) such as after pelvic RTx.

The most common cause of VVF in developing countries is obstructed labour, due to ischaemic necrosis of the anterior vaginal wall. [26]

VVF can be evaluated using *methylene blue 3-swab test*:

- Introduce 3 gauze swabs into the vagina via speculum inserted top, middle and bottom
- Catheterise patient and introduce methylene blue into bladder
- Remove catheter and ask patient to walk around for 30 minutes
- Swabs are removed and inspected – if any are stained blue this implies fistula; which swab is blue can give clue as to where fistula is located.

Imaging may include CTU and/or cystogram.

Small fistulae may heal with six weeks of urinary diversion (catheter +/- bilateral nephrostomies); unlikely, however, if cause is previous RTx.

Surgical Management

Options for repair of VVF are:

- Abdominal with omental flap interposition
- Vaginal with Martius fat pad interposition.

Success rates between the two techniques are comparable. [27]

Abdominal repair is associated with greater length of in-patient stay and morbidity; however, it preserves vaginal depth.

Vaginal repair has a lower associated morbidity and risk of ureteric injury; however, a greater risk of vaginal shortening.

If VVF is complex, multiple or failed reconstruction, patient may need ileal conduit urinary diversion or neobladder formation as last resort surgical options.

OTHER FISTULAE

The most common cause of colovesical fistulae is diverticular disease (colon cancer second most).

CT imaging should reveal air in the bladder, diverticulosis, with an area of thickened bladder next to a loop of thickened bowel (confirm findings with cystoscopy).

Vesicouterine fistulae occur most commonly after lower segment Caesarean section.

If fertility is not important to the patient, proceed to hysterectomy. Fertility preserving options include observation, cystoscopy and fulguration of fistula tract, repair with interposition of omental flap.

PELVIC ORGAN PROLAPSE

AETIOLOGY

The congenital causes of POP include:

- Connective tissue disorders e.g. Ehlers–Dahlos syndrome
- Spina bifida.

The acquired causes of POP include:

- Previous vaginal surgery (prolapse repair, colposuspension, hysterectomy)
- Obesity, chronic cough/constipation
- Previous vaginal delivery
- Low oestrogen levels.

Anterior wall prolapse is herniation of bladder (cystocoele) or urethra (urethrocoele).

Posterior wall prolapse is protrusion of rectum (rectocoele) or peritoneum (enterocoele).

Middle compartment prolapse includes uterine prolapse or procidentia (entire uterus).

CLASSIFICATION

POP quantification (POPQ) is a validated system which allows standardisation of descriptions of POP by measuring distances between defined anatomical points and the hymen.

The ICS has a staging of POP which is based on the POPQ (Table 4).

The *Baden and Walker system* provides a practical alternative classification tool (Table 5).

Table 4 – ICS staging of pelvic organ prolapse [28]

Stage	Leading Edge of POP in Relation to Hymen	Description
0	< -3cm	No POP
1	< -1cm	POP > 1cm above hymen
2	≤ -1cm and ≥ 1cm	POP between 1cm above and below hymen
3	> 1cm and < 2cm	POP > 1cm below hymen, no vaginal eversion
4		Complete vaginal eversion

Table 5 – Baden and Walker classification of pelvic organ prolapse [28]

Grade	Description
0	No prolapse
1	Descent halfway to the hymen
2	Descent to hymen
3	Descent halfway past the hymen
4	Maximal descent/eversion

DIAGNOSTIC EVALUATION

Patient History

The history should enquire regarding symptoms of:

- Vaginal pressure/bulge/heaviness or need for manual reduction
- Positional variation (i.e. worse when standing)
- Urinary dysfunction (retention, incontinence, frequency)
- Bowel dysfunction.

Consider requesting patient to complete validated questionnaire prior to clinic consultation, such as ICIQ-SF for incontinence, and bladder diary.

Patient Examination

Examination of the abdomen to evaluate for organomegaly, scars or palpable bladder.

Complete pelvic examination in the presence of female chaperone.

Undertake pelvic examination in standing, lithotomy and left lateral position (Sim's speculum):

- Retract anterior wall to visualise posterior compartment prolapse
- Retract posterior wall to demonstrate anterior/middle compartment prolapse
- Undertake cough test for SUI.

Perform urinalysis (send MSU for culture as appropriate), record PVR.

Consider MRI scan for select cases or surgical planning.

MANAGEMENT

Conservative

Counsel patient carefully in presence of community continence nurse.

Consider weight loss, moderate exercise, treating cough/constipation and supervised PFMT; treat vaginal atrophy where appropriate.

Refer patient to urogynaecologist.

Vaginal pessary is an option – individually fitted and changed every 3–6 months, where examination must be undertaken to check for vaginal erosion or ulceration.

Surgical

Prior to active intervention, the patient should be discussed at the local pelvic-floor MDT.

There are many different approaches depending on the underlying POP pathology.

For uterine prolapse consider hysterectomy (abdominal/vaginal) or sacro-hysteropexy if the patient wishes to preserve their uterus.

Repair may be with primary colposuspension.

REFERENCES

1. Nayar C, Kalsi V, Hamid R, et al. (2018). In: Arya M, Shergill IS, Fernando HS, et al., *Viva Practice for the FRCS (Urol) and Postgraduate Urology Examinations*, CRC Press, London.
2. Chai TC, Steers WD (1996). Neurophysiology of micturition and continence. *Urologic Clinics*, *23*(2), 221–236.
3. Reynard J, Brewster S, Biers S, et al. (2019). Neuropathic bladder. In: *Oxford Handbook of Urology*, fourth edition, Oxford University Press, Oxford.
4. Park JM, Bloom DA, McGuire EJ (1997). The guarding reflex revisited. *British Journal of Urology*, *80*(6), 940–945.
5. Blok B, Castro-Diaz D, Del Popolo G, et al. (2024). EAU Guidelines: Neuro-urology. Available at: https://d56bochluxqnz.cloudfront.net/documents/full-guideline/EAU-Guidelines-on-Neuro-Urology-2024.pdf [last accessed on 20 August 2024].
6. Fowler CJ (1999). Neurological disorders of micturition and their treatment. *Brain*, *122*(7), 1,213–1,231.
7. Stocchi F, Carbone A, Inghilleri M, et al. (1997). Urodynamic and neurophysiological evaluation in Parkinson's disease and multiple system atrophy. *Journal of Neurology, Neurosurgery & Psychiatry*, *62*(5), 507–511.
8. Karlsson AK (1999). Autonomic dysreflexia. *Spinal Cord*, *37*(6), 383–391.
9. Krassioukov A, Warburton DE, Teasell R, et al. (2009). A systematic review of the management of autonomic dysreflexia after spinal cord injury. *Archives of Physical Medicine and Rehabilitation*, *90*(4), 682–695.
10. British Association of Urological Surgeons. Available at: https://www.baus.org.uk/_userfiles/pages/files/Patients/Leaflets/ICIQ-UI.pdf [last accessed 10 June 2020].
11. Chevalier F, Fernandez-Lao C, Cuesta-Vargas AI (2014). Normal reference values of strength in pelvic floor muscle of women: a descriptive and inferential study. *BMC Women's Health*, *14*(1), 143.
12. Harding CK, Lapitan MC, Arlandis S, et al. (2024). EAU Guidelines: Non-neurogenic Female Lower Urinary Tract Symptoms. Available at: https://d56bochluxqnz.cloudfront.net/documents/full-guideline/EAU-Guidelines-on-Non-neurogenic-Female-LUTS-2024.pdf [last accessed 18 August 2024].
13. NICE (2019). Guidelines: Urinary incontinence and pelvic organ prolapse in women: management. Available at: https://www.nice.org.uk/guidance/ng123/resources/urinary-incontinence-and-pelvic-organ-prolapse-in-women-management-pdf-66141657205189 [last accessed 25 August 2024].

14. Novara G, Galfano A, Secco S, et al. (2008). A systematic review and meta-analysis of randomized controlled trials with antimuscarinic drugs for overactive bladder. *European Urology, 54*(4), 740–764.
15. Richardson K, Fox C, Maidment I, et al. (2018). Anticholinergic drugs and risk of dementia: case-control study. *BMJ, 361*, k1315.
16. Gray SL, Anderson ML, Dublin S, et al. (2015). Cumulative use of strong anticholinergics and incident dementia: a prospective cohort study. *JAMA Internal Medicine, 175*(3), 401–407.
17. Gratzke C, van Maanen R, Chapple C, et al. (2018). Long-term Safety and Efficacy of Mirabegron and Solifenacin in Combination Compared with Monotherapy in Patients with Overactive Bladder: A Randomised, Multicentre Phase 3 Study SYNERGY II. *European Urology, 74*(4), 501–509.
18. Cruz F, Herschorn S, Aliotta P, et al. (2011). Efficacy and safety of onabotulinumtoxinA in patients with urinary incontinence due to neurogenic detrusor overactivity: a randomised, double-blind, placebo-controlled trial. *European Urology, 60*(4), 742–750.
19. Nitti VW, Dmochowski R, Herschorn S, et al. (2013). OnabotulinumtoxinA for the treatment of patients with overactive bladder and urinary incontinence: results of a phase 3, randomized, placebo controlled trial. *Journal of Urology, 189*(6), 2,186–2,193.
20. Amundsen CL, Richter HE, Menefee SA, et al. (2016). OnabotulinumtoxinA vs Sacral Neuromodulation on Refractory Urgency Urinary Incontinence in Women. *JAMA, 316*(13), 1,366–1,374.
21. Blaivas JG, Olsson CA (1988). Stress incontinence: classification and surgical approach. *Journal of Urology, 139*(4), 727–731.
22. Freitas AMI, Mentula M, Rahkola-Soisalo P, et al. (2020). Tension-Free Vaginal Tape Surgery versus Polyacrylamide Hydrogel Injection for Primary Stress Urinary Incontinence: A Randomised Clinical Trial. *Journal of Urology, 203*(2), 372–378.
23. Albo ME, Richter HE, Brubaker L, et al. (2007). Burch Colposuspension versus Fascial Sling to Reduce Urinary Stress Incontinence. *New England Journal of Medicine, 356*(21), 2,143–2,155.
24. Abrams P, Constable LD, Cooper D, et al. (2021). Outcomes of a Noninferiority Randomised Controlled Trial of Surgery for Men with Urodynamic Stress Incontinence After Prostate Surgery (MASTER). *European Urology, 79*(6), 812–823.
25. Lim CS, Abrams P (1995). The Abrams-Griffiths nomogram. *World Journal of Urology, 13*(1), 34–39.
26. Romanzi LJ, Groutz A, Blaivas JG (2000). Urethral diverticulum in women: diverse presentations resulting in diagnostic delay and mismanagement. *Journal of Urology, 164*(2), 428–433.

27. Wall LL (2006). Obstetric vesicovaginal fistula as an international public-health problem. *Lancet, 368*(9,542), 1,201–1,209.
28. Persu C, Chapple CR, Cauni V, et al. (2011). Pelvic Organ Prolapse Quantification System (POP–Q) – a new era in pelvic prolapse staging. *Journal of Medicine and Life, 4*(1), 75.

BLADDER DYSFUNCTION & GYNAECOLOGICAL ASPECTS OF UROLOGY MCQS

1. *Where do the pre-ganglionic fibres of the sympathetic nerves to the bladder synapse with the post-ganglionic fibres?*
   A) Hypogastric plexus
   B) Inferior mesenteric plexus
   C) Superior mesenteric plexus
   D) Plexus of Raschkow
   E) Iliac plexus

2. *Where do the cell bodies of the pudendal nerve lie?*
   A) Onuf's nucleus
   B) Golgi nucleus
   C) Lateral geniculate nucleus
   D) Edinger–Westphal nucleus
   E) Hypogastric nucleus

3. *Via which ascending tracts do afferent nerves from the bladder carry information to the pontine micturition centre?*
   A) Corticospinal
   B) Tectospinal
   C) Spinothalamic
   D) Spinotectal
   E) Dorsolateral tract

4. *What is the most common UDS finding in MS patients with LUTS?*
   A) DetSD
   B) Detrusor underactivity
   C) Obstruction
   D) Poor compliance
   E) Detrusor overactivity

5. *What is the most common stimulus resulting in autonomic dysreflexia in a patient with a cervical spinal cord injury?*
   A) Faecal impaction
   B) Urine retention
   C) Peripheral pain/minor trauma
   D) UTI
   E) Urolithiasis

6. In terms of the benefit on number of micturitions and incontinence episodes, which treatment arms did the SYNERGY II Trial compare?

    A) (mirabegron) vs. (oxybutynin)
    B) (mirabegron) vs. (solifenacin)
    C) (mirabegron) vs. (solifenacin) vs. (oxybutynin)
    D) (mirabegron) vs. (solifenacin) vs. (mirabegron + solifenacin)
    E) (mirabegron) vs. (solifenacin) vs. (mirabegron + oxybutynin)

7. Which of the following is the most functionally relevant M-receptor in the bladder for detrusor muscle contractions?

    A) M1
    B) M2
    C) M3
    D) M4
    E) M5

8. Which of the following does BOTOX cleave off SNARE proteins to prevent the exocytosis of acetylcholine in its treatment of OAB/DO?

    A) ACH-15
    B) ACH-25
    C) SNAP-15
    D) SNAP-25
    E) SNAP-35

9. What is the correct starting dose for duloxetine to treat stress urinary incontinence?

    A) 20mg BD
    B) 200mg BD
    C) 10mg BD
    D) 100mg BD
    E) 1g BD

10. Which of the following is the correct minimum regimen as per NICE for pelvic-floor muscle training to manage stress urinary incontinence, before clinic follow-up?

    A) 6 contractions, twice daily, for ≥ 3 months
    B) 6 contractions, thrice daily, for ≥ 3 months
    C) 8 contractions, twice daily, for ≥ 3 months
    D) 8 contractions, thrice daily, for ≥ 3 months
    E) None of the above

11. *In artificial urethral sphincter insertion to treat women with SUI who have failed previous surgical intervention, where should the device reservoir be placed?*

    A) Rectovesical pouch
    B) Posterior rectus canal
    C) Rectouterine pouch
    D) Pouch of Douglas
    E) Space of Retzius

12. *Which of the following artificial urethral sphincter devices is the only one approved by the Food and Drug Administration (FDA)?*

    A) AMS 600
    B) AMS 800
    C) Br-SL-AS 604
    D) Br-SL-AS 904
    E) Zephyr ZS375

13. *Regarding the artificial urethral sphincter, which of the following is the constant circumferential pressure to compress the urethra usually set at?*

    A) 1–10cm H_2O
    B) 21–30cm H_2O
    C) 41–50cm H_2O
    D) 61–70cm H_2O
    E) 81–90cm H_2O

14. *What does a Valsalva leak-point pressure of < 60cm H_2O suggest?*

    A) Detrusor failure
    B) Intrinsic sphincter deficiency
    C) Urethral hypermobility
    D) DetSD
    E) Equivocal

15. *Which of the following bacteria is most commonly found in infections of artificial urethral sphincter devices?*

    A) E.coli
    B) S.aureus
    C) S.epidermidis
    D) Klebsiella
    E) Pseudomonas

16. *Where does a Martius labial fat flap obtain its blood supply from?*
    A) Internal pudendal artery
    B) External pudendal artery
    C) Both internal and external pudendal arteries
    D) Vaginal artery
    E) Artery to labia majora

17. *Which of the following conditions predisposes female patients to pelvic organ prolapse?*
    A) Ehlers–Dahlos syndrome
    B) Brown syndrome
    C) Cogan syndrome
    D) Osgood–Schlatter syndrome
    E) Kimmelstiel–Wilson syndrome

18. *On the Modified Oxford Grading System to evaluate pelvic-floor muscle strength, which of the following grades is defined as "weak"?*
    A) 0
    B) 1
    C) 2
    D) 3
    E) 4

19. *Which of the following is absorbed by the clammed bowel segment in augmentation cystoplasty, whose breakdown causes hyperchloraemic metabolic acidosis?*
    A) Hydrogen chloride
    B) Sodium chloride
    C) Potassium chloride
    D) Sodium bicarbonate
    E) Ammonium chloride

20. *Which of the following is the most common substance used to make synthetic mesh for surgical treatment of SUI?*
    A) Silicone
    B) Polypropylene
    C) Dacron
    D) Polyester
    E) Mersilene

STATION 8
ANDROLOGY & BPH

PROSTATE ANATOMY AND DEVELOPMENT

ARTERIAL SUPPLY

Internal iliac artery

→ anterior branch → inferior vesical artery → branches to the prostate

From the urethral group of arteries arise *Flock's* (1 and 11 o'clock) and *Badenoch's* (5 and 7 o'clock) arteries to supply the transitional zone of the prostate.

Image 1 – Arterial supply to prostate gland

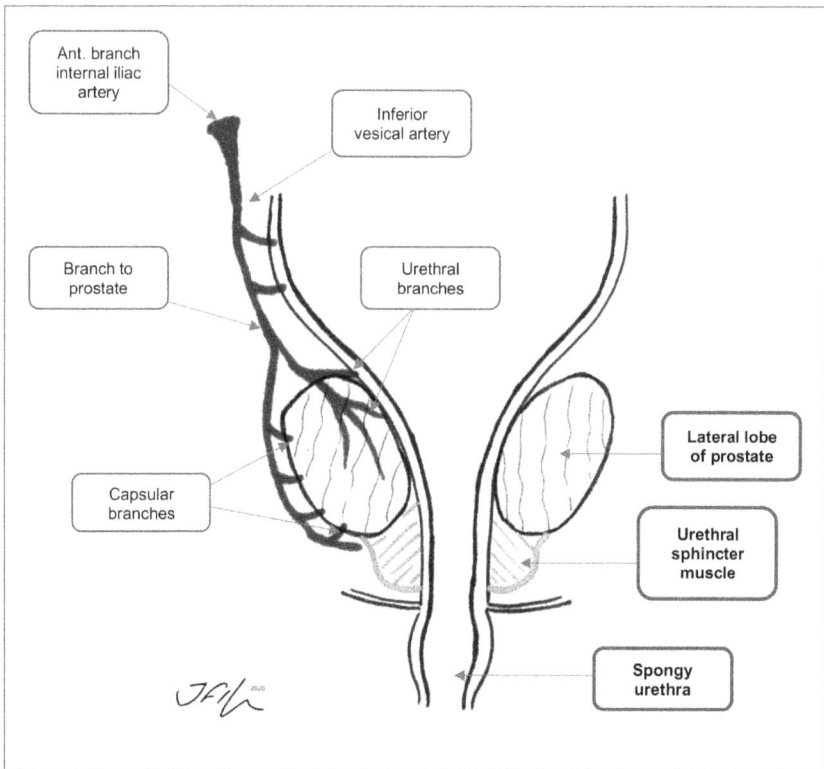

VENOUS DRAINAGE

Via the peri-prostatic venous plexus (which also receives the deep dorsal vein of the penis)

→ drains into internal iliac vein   → ipsilateral common iliac vein

LYMPHATIC DRAINAGE

Lymphatic drainage of the prostate is mainly to the obturator LN and subsequently internal iliac chain; there is also communication with external iliac, presacral, and the para-aortic LN.

Image 2 – Lymphatic drainage of prostate gland

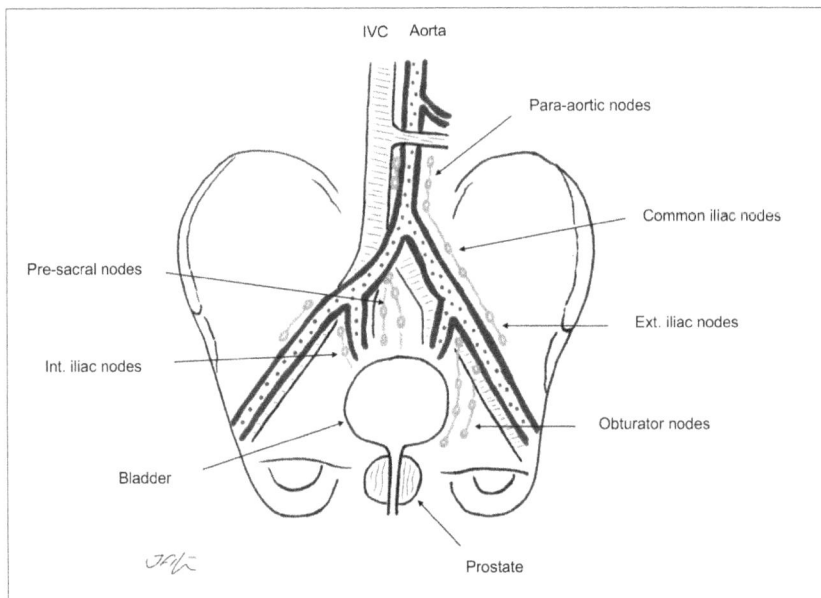

EMBRYOLOGY OF PROSTATE

Dual embryological origin – central zone derived from mesonephric duct, rest of prostate from the urogenital sinus.

At approximately 16 weeks gestation it arises under direct influence of 5-DHT.

ZONAL ANATOMY

McNeal described zones of the prostate from pathology specimens; however, the prostate is often described anatomically using lobes (anterior, median, posterior and 2 lateral) (see Table 1). [1]

Image 3 – Zonal anatomy of prostate gland

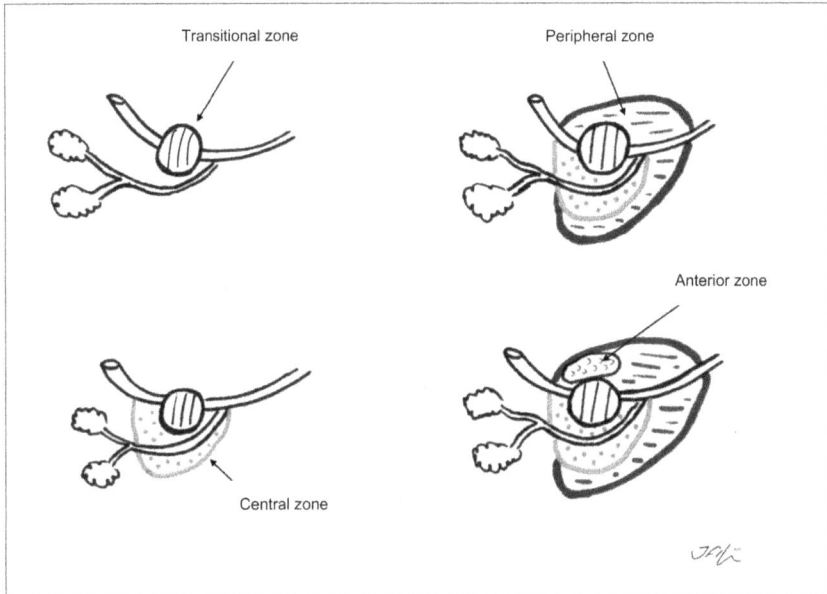

Table 1 – McNeal's zones of the prostate

McNeal Zone		Description
Peripheral zone	≤ 70% of glandular tissues	Site of origin for 70–80% of prostate cancers
Central zone	25% of glandular tissue	Zone surrounding ejaculatory ducts, < 5% cancers start here
Transition zone	10% of glandular tissue	Site of origin of BPH tissue changes
Anterior fibromuscular stroma	Approximately 5%	No glandular components, made of muscle + fibrous tissue

PHYSIOLOGY OF BPH

BPE is characterised by an increase in epithelial and stromal cell numbers in the peri-urethral area of the prostate (i.e. transition zone).

BPH describes the histological findings of suspected BPE.

Combination of increased cell proliferation (early phase) and reduction in apoptosis (latter phase).

In established BPH, cell proliferation slows down and programmed cell death is impaired.

Normal prostatic stromal tissue has a substantial smooth muscle component (~50%); however, in BPH the proportion of this is less (~25%).

The symptoms and effects of BPE are caused by two main components:

- *Static*, mediated by volume effect of BPE
- *Dynamic*, due to α1-adrenoreceptor mediated prostatic smooth muscle contraction.

This is the rationale for α-adrenoreceptor blocker treatment (e.g. tamsulosin).

Role of Androgens in BPH

Testosterone can bind to androgen receptors directly, or may be converted to the more potent form DHT.

This conversion is mediated by the enzyme 5AR which can be:

- *Type 1* (extra-prostatic, in liver and skin) or
- *Type 2* (found exclusively on nuclear membrane of stromal cells (not epithelial cells).

Finasteride inhibits type-2 5AR only, reducing serum DHT by 70% and prostatic DHT by 80%. [2]

Dutasteride inhibits both types 1 and 2 5AR, reducing serum DHT by 95% and prostatic DHT by 94%. [3]

The difference in their reductions of DHT does not translate into clinically significant differences in the efficacy of the drugs.

Testosterone diffuses into prostate stromal and epithelial cells:

- Within epithelial cells it binds directly to the androgen receptor
- Within stromal cells the majority binds to type-2 (5AR), is then converted to DHT which binds to the androgen receptor (with greater affinity and potency).

The androgen receptor/testosterone or androgen receptor/DHT complexes bind in the nucleus to induce transcription of androgen-dependent genes and protein synthesis (Figure 1).

Figure 1 – Action of testosterone and DHT in prostate epithelial cell

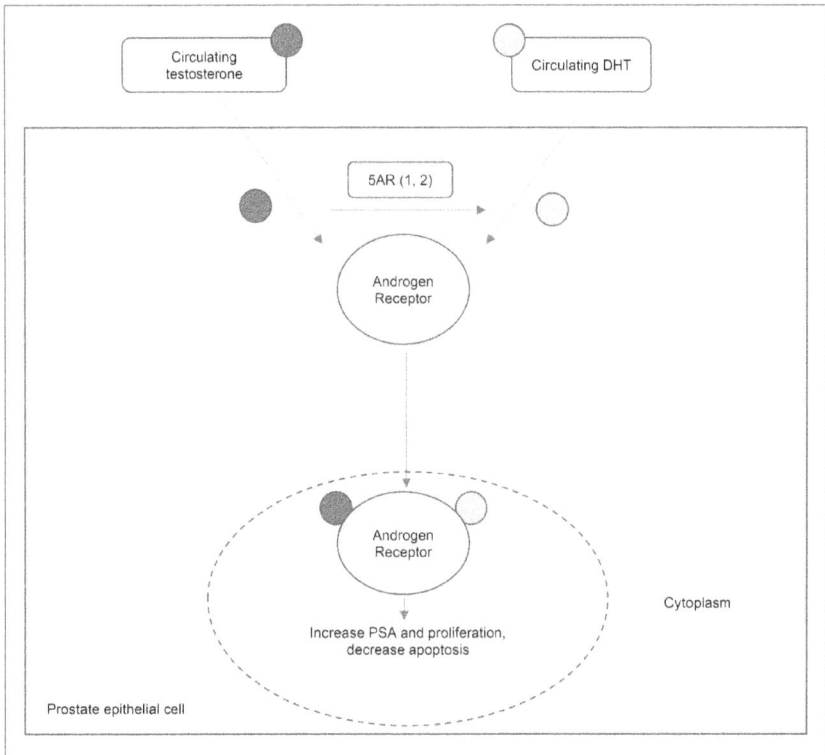

EJACULATORY DISORDERS

RETROGRADE EJACULATION

Retrograde ejaculation involves failure of bladder neck contraction causing retrograde flow of semen into bladder on ejaculation.

Acquired causes of retrograde ejaculation include:

- Iatrogenic anatomical disruption, e.g. TURP, BNI
- Drugs, e.g. α-blockers (reversible), SSRIs, risperidone
- Neurological, e.g. diabetic neuropathy, retro-peritoneal dissection.

Congenital causes of retrograde ejaculation include spina bifida.

DIAGNOSTIC EVALUATION

The key factors to enquire about in the patient history include:

- Dry ejaculate at orgasm followed by noticing cloudy urine on voiding
- Assessing for risk factors as listed above
- Infertility.

Patient examination may be unremarkable.

Perform semen analysis, which will reveal low ejaculate volume < 1mL.

A post-orgasm urine examination reveals sperm in specimen to confirm the diagnosis.

MANAGEMENT

Treatment is only needed if patient is wishing to restore natural fertility.

Reversible causes (such as α-blocker medication) should be addressed.

Medical Treatment

Medication can be used to try to close the bladder neck.

Sympathomimetics (α-adrenergics) such as pseudoephedrine can be given 7–10 days prior to planned ejaculation (often in view of female ovulation time).

Imipramine (tricyclic antidepressant) may also be used.

Sperm Retrieval

If medical therapy fails, sperm can be retrieved from alkalinised post-ejaculate urine, as acidic urine is thought to be spermicidal.

Patient must take sodium bicarbonate orally the night before and on the morning of producing sample.

Patient is asked to empty their bladder and then masturbate; afterwards a post-ejaculation urine sample is collected and delivered to the laboratory.

The lab will centrifuge the sample – retrieved sperm can also be used for IVF or IUI.

PREMATURE EJACULATION

There is no validated or accurate definition for diagnosing premature ejaculation.

The *International Society for Sexual Medicine* defines this as a male sexual dysfunction in which ejaculation always or almost always occurs within 1 minute of penetration. [4]

Premature ejaculation is characterised by:

- Inability to delay ejaculation during sexual activity
- Resulting in negative personal consequences/low satisfaction with sexual relationship.

The aetiology of premature ejaculation is relatively unknown.

Premature ejaculation can be broadly classified into 4 sub-types:

- *Lifelong*
- *Acquired*, due to psychological/relationship problems, performance anxiety
- *Variable*, considered a normal variation of sexual function
- *Subjective*, stemming from cultural or misperceptions.

DIAGNOSTIC EVALUATION

The key factors to evaluate in the patient history include:

- Determining whether the premature ejaculation is lifelong or acquired
- Impact on patient QOL/relationships/mood
- Estimated time from penetration to ejaculation.

Complete chaperoned examination of patient's external genitalia, which is likely to be unremarkable.

Routine laboratory tests are not recommended.

MANAGEMENT

Reassure patient that premature ejaculation is not an uncommon problem to occur in a man's life.

Psychosexual counselling may be beneficial and they should be signposted to consulting this service.

Behavioural Strategies

The *Masters and Johnson squeeze technique* involves:

- Patient being stimulated to the point at which they feel like they are about to ejaculate
- Patient or partner should then apply firm pressure to the base of penis for 30 seconds
- Once urge to ejaculate subsides, sexual activity can be resumed.

The *stop–start technique* involves:

- Patient being stimulated to the point at which they feel like they are about to ejaculate
- Stop sexual stimulation for about 30 seconds until control is regained
- Repeat the stop–start technique several times before allowing orgasm to occur.

Pharmacological

SSRI drugs can be used on demand to treat premature ejaculation.

Serotonin as a neurotransmitter is believed to exert an inhibitory role on ejaculation.

Dapoxetine is the only licensed SSRI for such use in the UK and is recommended first line (EAU 2024); other agents such as sertraline, fluoxetine or paroxetine are unlicensed uses.

Dapoxetine has a short half-life (≤ 24 hours) and patient should be counselled:

- Not to use drug daily, but only on PRN basis
- Take drug approximately 1 hour prior to sexual activity
- Starting dose is 30mg, which can be increased up to 60mg/day.

Dapoxetine may increase risk of ED and therefore concomitant PDE5i use may be required.

Off-label SSRI (e.g. fluoxetine) as second-line therapy can be given if daily medication is required (EAU 2024); however, prescribe with caution if associated depressive disorder or suicidal ideation.

Alternatives include topical (spray or cream) lidocaine or prilocaine, to reduce penile sensitivity.

ANEJACULATION

The complete absence of antegrade/retrograde ejaculation is termed anejaculation.

This condition can be caused by:

- Spinal cord injury
- Congenital bilateral absence of vas deferens (CBAVD) seen in CF
- Retro-peritoneal LN dissection.

Semen can be obtained using a Seager electro-ejaculator (rectal probe stimulation) or retrieval can be undertaken to be used for IVF and IUI.

VASECTOMY

A patient requesting vasectomy should be seen in the routine general urology clinic.

The key factors to evaluate in the patient history include:

- Current family and future family plans
- Awareness of alternative methods of contraception for himself and partner
- Previous scrotal surgery (might make surgery under local anaesthesia challenging)
- Understanding that intervention is permanent and that reversal is not available on the NHS.

Ensure that on chaperoned patient examination you can feel both vas deferens easily – if you are unable to, the patient may benefit from having the procedure under GA.

If patient is keen to proceed, the following risks/side-effects must be discussed:

- Early failure rate (1 in 250)
- Late failure rate (1 in 2,000) due to re-canalisation
- Chronic testicular pain ($\leq$ 5%)
- Bruising/haematoma requiring drainage/infection
- Not reversible on the NHS.

After the vasectomy is completed, the patient must continue to use barrier contraception.

Sperm should continue to be cleared by normal ejaculations (> 20 ejaculations are recommended).

After $\geq$ 12 weeks from vasectomy, the patient is required to provide a semen sample for analysis after a minimum of 3 days of abstinence.

A single azoospermic sample after 12 weeks is sufficient to give all clear to have unprotected sex. [5]

For those not azoospermic at the first test sample, 95% will be at repeat sampling 6 weeks later.

Special clearance can be given 28 weeks post-vasectomy, provided < 10^5/mL of non-motile sperm.

> **VIVA** You may be asked to consent a patient for vasectomy in your FRCS (Urol) viva – you would be expected to know the exact figures for the risks of early and late failure, as well as instructions for post-procedural use of barrier contraception and when to deliver the semen sample for being granted the all-clear status. I recommend you mention you would provide the patient with written information and encourage them to read this and reflect, before confirming their decision to go ahead.

VASECTOMY REVERSAL

Approximately 6% of men will request a reversal of vasectomy. [6]

The surgery requires micro-apposition of the vas ends:

- Multi-layer vaso-vasostomy
- Single-layer vaso-vasostomy
- Inguinal vaso-vasostomy (e.g. if vas obstructed within inguinal canal from hernia repair)
- Epididymo-vaso-vasostomy.

Key principles include precise end-to-end approximation (prevent sperm leakage and granuloma formation) and non-tension (compromise blood supply).

A sample of sperm fluid should be taken from the proximal vas and analysed.

Overall patency rates are high ($\leq$ 90%). [7]

Success rates depend on time interval since vasectomy was performed (Table 2).

If reversal is not successful, patient can alternatively undergo sperm-retrieval procedures.

Table 2 – Patency and pregnancy rates categorised by time since vasectomy [8]

Time from Vasectomy (Years)	Patency Rate (%)	Pregnancy Rate (%)
< 3	97	76
3–8	88	53
9–14	79	44
$\geq$ 15	71	30

ERECTILE DYSFUNCTION

PENILE ANATOMY

ARTERIAL SUPPLY

> Internal iliac artery (anterior branch) ➔ internal pudendal artery ➔ common penile artery (main supply)

Accessory supply may derive from branches of external iliac, obturator, vesical and femoral arteries.

The main branches of the common penile artery are:

- *Cavernous:* involved in tumescence of corpora cavernosa (via helicine branches, which become dilated and straight during erection)
- *Dorsal:* provides engorgement of penis during erection
- *Bulbar:* supplies bulb and corpus spongiosum.

VENOUS DRAINAGE

Venous drainage from the three corpora:

- Originates in venules and travels between tunica and peripheral sinusoids
- Forms the sub-tunical venular plexus before exiting as emissary veins
- Drains into deep dorsal vein (dorsally), circumflex vein (laterally) peri-urethral veins (ventrally)
- Ultimately enters the vesical and prostatic plexuses.

The *deep dorsal vein of the penis* runs directly beneath the superficial dorsal vein, separated from it by the deep fascia of penis, and drains the glans and corpora cavernosa.

The superficial drainage system (lying outside Buck's fascia) drains the prepuce and skin of shaft.

Smaller superficial veins merge on the dorsolateral aspect of the penis near root of penis to form the *superficial dorsal vein of the penis*, which drains into saphenous veins.

INNERVATION

Autonomic

Sympathetic nerves (T11–L2) and parasympathetic nerves (S2–4) join to form pelvic plexus.

Cavernosal nerves are branches of the pelvic plexus that innervate penis:

- Parasympathetic supply causes erection
- Sympathetic supply causes ejaculation and detumescence.

Somatic

Sensory (afferent) information travels via dorsal penile and pudendal nerves to enter cord S2–4.

Onuf's nucleus (S2–4) is the somatic centre for efferent innervation of ischio- and bulbocavernosus muscles of the penis.

CROSS-SECTIONAL VIEW

Image 4 – Cross-sectional anatomical view of penis [9]

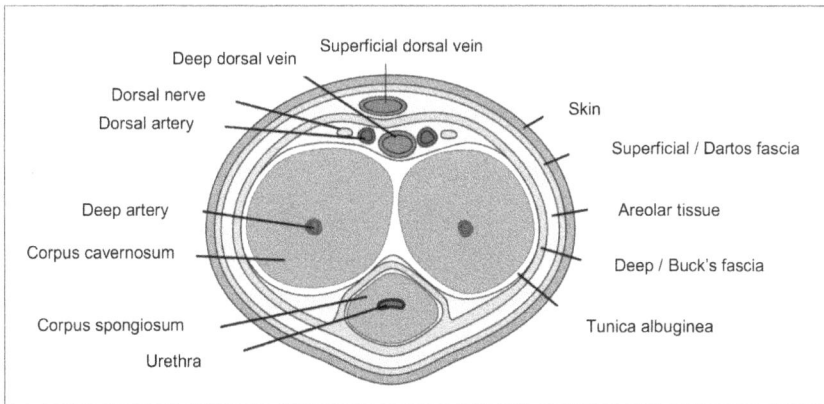

PHYSIOLOGY OF ERECTION

In the flaccid state, the smooth muscle of the arteriolar walls is tonically contracted, allowing only small amount of arterial flow into cavernous spaces.

Subsequently audio/tactile/visual stimuli create neuroendocrine signals from the brain.

These activate the autonomic nuclei of the spinal erection centre (T11–L2) and (S2–4).

Signals are conveyed via cavernosal nerves to erectile tissue of corpora cavernosa, releasing neurotransmitters from the cavernous nerve terminals.

This results in smooth muscle relaxation, activating the veno-occlusive mechanism and triggering:

- Dilatation of arterioles/arteries by increased blood flow
- Trapping of incoming blood by expanding sinusoids
- Compression of sub-tunical venular plexuses (reduces venous outflow)
- Stretching tunica to capacity which encloses emissary veins (reduces venous outflow)
- Rise in intra-cavernous pressure (e.g. 100mmHg) – *full erection* phase
- Further pressure rise due to ischiocavernous muscle contraction – *rigid erection* phase.

There are five distinct phases of penile erection that have been demonstrated.

Detumescence has initial, slow and fast phases.

Table 3 – Phases of erection

Phase	Term (Phase)	Description
0	Flaccid	Cavernosal muscle contracted
		Sinusoids empty
		Minimal arterial flow
1	Latent (filling)	Increased pudendal artery flow (peak flow ~25mL/min at end of latent phase)
		Penile elongation
2	Tumescent	Rising intra-cavernosal pressure
		Erection forming
3	Full erection	Increased cavernosal pressure
		Penis becomes full erect
4	Rigid erection	Further increases in pressure (peak intra-corporeal pressure, minimal blood flow)
		Ischiocavernous muscle contraction
5	Detumescent	Sympathetic discharge continues after ejaculation
		Smooth muscle contraction/vasoconstriction
		Reduced arterial flow, blood out from sinusoidal spaces

CAVERNOSAL SMOOTH MUSCLE

NO, VIP, PGE1 → decrease in calcium → RELAXATION (erection)

Following ejaculation, vasoconstriction (by sympathetic activity, endothelin, PGF2, cGMP breakdown) causes detumescence.

NA released from sympathetic nerve terminals acts on smooth muscle α-1 adrenoreceptors to raise intracellular calcium, helping maintain flaccidity.

NA, endothelin-1, PGF2 → increased calcium sensitivity → CONTRACTION (flaccidity)

Figure 2 – Secondary messenger pathways involved in erection

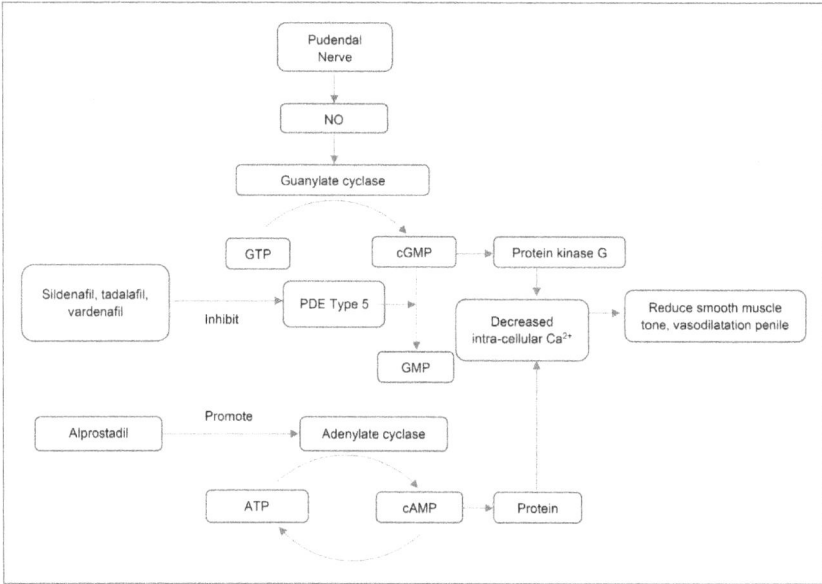

EJACULATION

Stimulation sends sensory information via pudendal nerve to lumbar sympathetic nuclei.

Sympathetic efferent signs via hypogastric nerve causing:

- Contraction of smooth muscle of epididymis, vas deferens, secretory glands
- Propelling spermatozoa and glandular secretions into prostatic urethra
- Closure of internal urethral sphincter and relaxation of extrinsic sphincter
- Rhythmic contraction of bulbocavernosus muscle for emission of ejaculate.

Average volume of ejaculate is 2–5mL.

AETIOLOGY OF ERECTILE DYSFUNCTION

There is a high prevalence and incidence of ED worldwide.

Incidence increases with age – complete ED incidence estimated in 70s (15%) and 80s (30–40%).

ED is divided into *primary psychogenic* vs. *primary organic* causes (although commonly mixed).

An organic cause is more likely in the following scenarios:

- Gradual onset (unless cause is obvious such as trauma/pelvic surgery)
- Loss of spontaneous/morning erections
- Intact libido with normal ejaculatory function
- Existing medical factors and older age groups.

ED can be a presenting symptom of underlying disease (Table 4).

Table 4 – Categorised causes of erectile dysfunction

Cause	Examples of Diseases
Vasculogenic	CVD, diabetes, hyperlipidaemia, smoking, obesity
Neurogenic	CKD, SCI, CVA, MS, Parkinson's, surgery/RTx to pelvis
Anatomical	Peyronie's, micropenis, phimosis
Hormonal	Hypogonadism, hypo-/hyperthyroid, high prolactin, high or low cortisol
Drug-induced	SSRIs, tricyclics, antipsychotics, alcohol, cocaine, β-blockers, thiazides
Trauma	Penile and pelvic fractures
Psychogenic	Anxiety, depression

There is consistent evidence for association between LUTS/BPH and ED in older men.

The most important factor associated with recovery of erections after RP is pre-operative potency.

DIAGNOSTIC EVALUATION

History

Patient should be seen in a dedicated ED clinic, in the presence of partner and ED specialist nurse.

A full sexual history should be taken, enquiring in particular about:

- Duration of onset of ED
- Whether morning erections are present or not
- Situational ED i.e. is it present on masturbation, does it vary depending on partner
- Screen for risk factors including full drug history/alcohol/smoking
- Psychosocial factors
- Concomitant presence of LUTS.

A validated questionnaire should be used to assess the severity of the ED (EAU 2024).

These are helpful in assessing domains of sexual function as well as impact of treatment.

The IIEF-5 questionnaire(Image 5) (abriged from the 15-item IIEF questionnaire) can be used and pertains to last 6 months of patient sex life. [10]

Image 5 – IIEF-5 questionnaire [10]

		Very low	Low	Moderate	High	Very high
1	How do you rate your **confidence** that you could get and keep an erection?	Very low 1	Low 2	Moderate 3	High 4	Very high 5
2	When you had erections with sexual stimulation, how often were your erections hard enough for penetration?	Almost never/never 1	A few times (much less than half the time) 2	Sometimes (about half the time) 3	Most times (much more than half the time) 4	Almost always/always 5
3	During sexual intercourse, **how often** were you able to maintain your erection after you had penetrated (entered) your partner?	Almost never/never 1	A few times (much less than half the time) 2	Sometimes (about half the time) 3	Most time (much more than half the time) 4	Almost always/always 5
4	During sexual intercourse, **how difficult** was it to maintain your erection to completion of intercourse?	Extremely difficult 1	Very difficult 2	Difficult 3	Slightly difficult 4	Not difficult 5
5	When you attempted sexual intercourse, how often was it satisfactory for you?	Almost never/never 1	A few times (much less than half the time) 2	Sometimes (about half the time) 3	Most times (much more than half the time) 4	Almost always/always 5

The overall score allows the severity of ED to be assessed and categorised objectively (Table 5).

Table 5 – Score categories for IIEF-5 questionnaire

Score	Severity
1–7	Severe
8–11	Moderate
12–16	Mild to moderate
17–21	Mild to moderate
22–25	No ED

The IIEF-5 questionnaire is also known as The Sexual Health Inventory for Men (SHIM).

Note that SHIM is not validated for use in ED associated with Peyronie's disease.

> **VIVA** You may be asked in your FRCS (Urol) viva to assess a patient with ED. A strong opening gambit would be: "I would see this patient in a dedicated ED clinic in the presence of my ED specialist nurse, preferably with the patient's partner present. Prior to entering the consultation room I would kindly ask him to complete an IIEF-5 questionnaire, and have his height, weight and BMI recorded. I would welcome him in the clinic room, introduce myself and take a focused sexual history…"

Examination

A full physical examination is mandatory with consent in the presence of a chaperone.

The following should all be assessed:

- Cardiovascular system: measure blood pressure, heart rate, BMI/waist circumference
- Genitalia: size of testes, phimosis, evidence of Peyronie's
- DRE of prostate: assess for BPH or PCa
- Development of secondary sexual characteristics.

Baseline Investigations

Baseline investigations will depend on the history and examination of the patient.

Blood tests that should be considered include:

- Fasting glucose, HBA1c and lipid profile
- Serum (free) early morning testosterone (if low then perform LH, FSH, SHBG)
- Serum prolactin
- PSA (if abnormal DRE).

Most patients with ED can be managed in the secondary care setting with no further tests than above.

Select patients may need specific diagnostic tests:

- Primary ED (not caused by organic disease or psychogenic)
- Young patients with pelvic/perineal trauma (may benefit from revascularisation)
- Pre-implantation of penile prosthesis
- Complex endocrine or psychiatric disorders
- Penile deformities.

Rigiscan Device

This provides nocturnal penile tumescence and rigidity testing.

Device containing two rings applied to penile tip and base, used to measure number/duration/rigidity of nocturnal erections.

This can help to differentiate between psychogenic and organic pathology.

A functional erectile mechanism is indicated by an erectile event of ≥ 60% rigidity recorded on tip of penis that lasts for ≥ 10 minutes. [11]

Penile Colour Doppler

Radiological investigation of choice if suspected underlying vascular cause for ED.

Intra-cavernosal PGE1 injection is given to induce erection, the blood flow is then measured to diagnose *arteriogenic, veno-occlusive* or *mixed vasculogenic* ED.

Peak systolic velocity should be > 30cm/s (if lower than this value, suggests arteriogenic ED).

End diastolic velocity < 5cm/s (if higher than this, suggests veno-occlusive ED).

Cavernosography

A cavernosogram should only be performed in patients who are being considered for vascular reconstruction surgery.

Cavernosography requires artificial erection followed by injection of contrast into penis.

Flow is maintained throughout imaging to demonstrate any venous leaks.

Penile arteriography is rarely performed due to advent of penile prostheses; however, contrast via pudendal artery is given before and after drug-induced erection.

Penile revascularisation surgery most commonly addresses internal pudendal artery stenosis.

MANAGEMENT

CONSERVATIVE

ED is often associated with modifiable/reversible risk factors (e.g. drugs, alcohol, high BMI).

These factors should be modified either before or during the time that specific therapies are used, including any relevant comorbidities that need optimising.

Testosterone Supplementation

Testosterone deficiency may be primary (primary testicular failure) or secondary (low LH/FSH).

Testosterone supplementation is effective but should only be given once other endocrinological causes for low testosterone have been ruled out.

Prior to prescribing testosterone, you should perform DRE, PSA, haematocrit, liver profile and LFT.

Testosterone supplementation is contraindicated in untreated PCa and unstable cardiac disease.

Testosterone can be given via oral/topical/IM routes.

Oral agents are rapidly absorbed by the gut and broken down in first pass of liver metabolism (i.e. poorly effective), unless testosterone undecanoate is used which enters the lymphatic system.

Intramuscular administration can result in high-peak/low-trough levels (weekly or 6-weekly dosing) which may lead to mood swings, in addition to potential discomfort at injection site.

PHOSPHODIESTERASE TYPE-5 INHIBITORS

NO enters smooth muscle cells to activate soluble guanylate cyclase which catalyses GTP ➔ cGMP.

cGMP facilitates smooth muscle relaxation (reduction in intracellular calcium) for erection.

cGMP is terminated when it is metabolised to inactive GMP, mediated by PDE5.

PDE5i therefore facilitate NO-induced smooth muscle relaxation by accumulation of cGMP, by preventing its breakdown to GMP.

Side-effects of PDE5i drugs include:

- Headache, flushing, dizziness,
- Nasal congestion
- Back pain.

PDE5i can be used in conjunction with testosterone supplementation.

Approximately 25% of patients do not respond to PDE5i drugs.

Use PDE5i as first-line therapy for the treatment of ED (EAU 2024). [11]

Options include sildenafil, tadalafil, vardenafil, avanafil.

Contraindications

PDE5i are contraindicated in patients taking nitrates – they result in cGMP accumulation and unpredictable falls in blood pressure.

If PDE5i is taken, the nitrate must be withheld at least for the length of the chosen PDE5i's half-life.

PDE5i can be used with other anti-hypertensives with caution.

PDE5i should <u>not</u> be used if recent MI/stroke ≤ 6 months, severe heart failure, unstable angina or angina during intercourse.

Sildenafil has a *severe*-rated severity interaction in the BNF with tamsulosin (risk of hypotension).

Sildenafil (Viagra®)

Sildenafil was the first PDE5i available on the market.

Used on demand, efficacy within 30–60 minutes which may be maintained for ≤ 12 hours.

Efficacy is reduced after heavy fatty meal due to delayed absorption.

Tadalafil (Cialis®)

Efficacy is maintained for 36 hours, not affected by food (no reduced bioavailability).

Tadalafil is the only PDE5i available for daily dosing, therefore may be preferable for spontaneity.

Can be used to treat male LUTS (preferable option if ED co-existing with LUTS).

Vardenafil (Levitra®)

Efficacy is reduced after heavy fatty meal due to delayed absorption.

Table 6 – Comparison of different PDE5i drugs

Drug	Dose (mg)	Modality	Half-life (Hours)	Onset of Action
Sildenafil	25, 50, 100	On demand	4–5	30 mins
Tadalafil	5, 10, 20	Daily (5) and on demand	17.5	30 mins (peak 120)
Vardenafil	5, 10, 20	On demand	4–5	30 mins

No trial has proven superior efficacy of any of the PDE5i drugs.

Drug choice will depend on patient preference regarding number of desired intercourses per week, need for short- vs. long-lasting medication and side-effects.

PDE5i failure should be confirmed only if patient fails to respond after $\geq$ 6 trials at maximum dosage, patient can then be offered daily dosing or second-line therapy.

IC_{50} (half maximal inhibitory concentration) refers to concentration of an antagonist that produces 50% of the maximum inhibitory effect of that antagonist (i.e. PDE5i is the antagonist).

Vardanafil's IC_{50} is 10x lower (i.e. the drug is more potent).

NHS Prescribing

The patent on sildenafil expired in 2019.

Sildenafil can be prescribed in England on the NHS to treat ED irrespective of underlying cause; however, only in its generic form (i.e. not Viagra®, which is considerably more expensive).

Viagra® can be prescribed only in context of select underlying conditions (e.g. diabetes, SCI).

Tadalafil is only available on NHS if patient meets specific criteria (e.g. MS, SCI).

VACUUM ERECTION DEVICE

Provide passive engorgement of corpora together with constrictor ring applied to base of penis.

Satisfaction rates $\leq$ 90%; most who discontinue do so within first 3 months.

Contraindicated in bleeding disorders or anti-coagulant therapy. To prevent skin necrosis the ring should be removed soon after intercourse.

INTRA-CAVERNOSAL INJECTIONS

Alprostadil can be delivered as injection into corpora cavernosa – patient must be suitably trained.

Caverject®/Viridal®Duo are available preparations; use as monotherapy in doses of 5–40µg.

Efficacy rates > 70% are reported.

Most common side-effect is penile pain which is self-limiting, others include priapism and fibrosis, and the development of Peyronie's should indicate stopping therapy indefinitely.

Most drop-outs occur within 3 months of commencing treatment.

EAU 2024 recommends intra-cavernosal injections as alternative first-line ED therapy. [11]

TOPICAL/INTRA-URETHRAL ALPROSTADIL

Alprostadil is a synthetic prostaglandin.

Can be provided as 500µg–1,000µg doses to be used on demand, administered as pellet via tiny stick into the urethra (MUSE®).

Efficacy lower than intra-cavernosal treatment (< 65%); however, may be preferable as less invasive, and can be augmented by use of constricting ring at penile base.

Local pain is the most common side-effect.

Similar preparation of alprostadil (Vitaros®) can be delivered as a cream into urethra (dose 300µ).

EAU 2024 recommends topical/intra-urethral alprostadil as alternative first-line ED therapy. [11]

PENILE PROSTHESES

Surgical implantation of a penile prosthesis should be considered in the following patients:

- Failure/unwilling/unable to consider first- and second-line treatment options
- Refractory ED with severe Peyronie's disease
- Penile fibrosis (e.g. after prolonged ischaemic priapism)
- Following penile trauma.

The available options are *malleable* or *inflatable* devices.

Malleable devices can be manually placed into erect or flaccid state.

Inflatable devices often preferred as they allow more natural erections to be obtained.

3-piece inflatable device consists of reservoir placed in retropubic space (auto-inflation is less likely) and filled with saline, pump placed in scrotum and pair of cylinders within the corpora of penis.

Satisfaction rates with penile prosthesis, regardless of the cause, are ≥ 90%.

The patient must be counselled that the implant will not give them an erection (i.e. a natural one) but rather a uniformly rigid penis on demand.

The *side-effects* of penile prosthesis surgery include:

- Infection, erosion, mechanical failure (< 5%)
- Glans droop (may require glanspexy).

Infection rate (< 5%) most commonly due to staphylococcal organisms; higher in diabetic patients and those taking steroid medications (≤ 50%).

Severe infection will require implant removal, and delaying reinsertion may increase fibrosis risk and complexity of re-do surgery.

The *Mulcahy technique* is a 7-step strategy wash-out system involving a series of antimicrobial agents and mechanical lavage of all spaces (reservoir space, corpora).

ED AFTER RADICAL PROSTATECTOMY

The use of pro-erectile drugs after RP is important in achieving post-operative erectile function.

Higher rates of erectile function recovery after RP have been shown in patient receiving any drug (therapeutic or prophylactic) for ED (penile rehabilitation).

PDE-5i are considered first line after RP – although such patients are considered poor responders.

More invasive options are intra-cavernosal injections (second line) and penile prostheses (third line).

MALE HYPOGONADISM

PATHOPHYSIOLOGY

Male hypogonadism can be considered:

- *Primary*, due to testicular failure (e.g. mumps orchitis, chemotherapy, RTx, trauma)
- *Secondary*, due to insufficient GnRH/FSH/LH (e.g. Kallmann syndrome, pituitary pathology)
- Androgen receptor insensitivity.

LOH is defined as a syndrome associated with advancing age, comprising both clinically specific symptoms as well as biochemical evidence of testosterone deficiency.

Ageing decreases the production of LHRH and LH, resulting in a decline in both number of Leydig cells and their sensitivity to LH.

LOH is associated with obesity, diabetes and overall poor health.

DIAGNOSTIC EVALUATION

History

Evaluate for the following common LOH symptoms in the patient history:

- ED along with reduced libido
- Lethargy, reduced exercise tolerance, poor concentration, change in mood, sleep disturbance
- Loss of muscle mass and hair
- Headache or visual disturbance may suggest a pituitary pathology.

Examination

Patient examination should be systematic and performed in the presence of a chaperone.

The following aspects should be assessed:

- BMI and waist circumference
- Evidence of hair loss and thinning
- Presence of gynaecomastia
- DRE
- Soft and small-volume testes (average testicular volume ~20mL).

BASELINE INVESTIGATIONS

Request bloods for LH/FSH, early-morning total testosterone (peak levels 7am–11am) and prolactin.

Testosterone upper and lower limits of normal vary in UK NHS labs, usually 6–27nmol/L.

Total testosterone < 12nmol/L is a reliable threshold to diagnose LOH (EAU 2024).

If testosterone is low (< 12nmol/L), EAU 2024 recommends confirming this low reading on two further separate occasions, prior to considering testosterone replacement therapy. [11]

Consider fasting glucose, HBA1c and lipid profile.

A baseline DEXA scan can be considered to assess BMD, due to risk of osteoporosis.

SHBG

If testosterone is low, consider measuring SHBG.

SHBG naturally binds approximately 45% of total circulating testosterone in healthy young men, which is tightly bound and not available for tissue use.

Bioavailable testosterone = (free testosterone ~2%) + (albumin-bound testosterone)

SHBG will increase with age, which reflects the natural fall in free testosterone.

SHBG levels can be affected by liver cirrhosis, hyperthyroidism, oestrogen use and HIV.

MANAGEMENT

Patients with symptomatic LOH (testosterone < 12nmol/L), without contraindications, are suitable candidates to be prescribed testosterone replacement therapy.

Contraindications to testosterone replacement therapy include:

- Active prostate or breast cancer (absolute)
- Men with active desire to father children (absolute)
- Elevated haematocrit (absolute)
- Uncontrolled congestive heart failure (absolute)
- Clinically significant BPH such as IPSS > 19 (relative)
- Family or personal history of VTE.

Prior to commencing testosterone replacement therapy, evaluate and document:

- DRE of prostate findings and baseline PSA
- Baseline lipid profile, LFT, UE, FBC + haematocrit
- Consider baseline DEXA scan if history of osteoporosis.

Follow-up monitoring protocols vary; EAU 2024 recommends measuring serum testosterone at 3, 6 and 12 months after starting replacement therapy, and thereafter annually.

In addition, annual DRE, PSA, FBC, LFT, lipid profile and blood pressure monitoring are advisable. [12]

The most common abnormality is raised haematocrit which will settle if testosterone replacement therapy is stopped (the highest risk of this is noted with IM administration).

After cessation of TRT, the symptoms related to its deficiency are likely to return.

Methods of Delivery

Methods available for delivering testosterone replacement therapy are categorised in Table 7.

Oral formulations are limited by poor bioavailability, as they are strongly dependent on dietary fat content, and are therefore not routinely recommended.

Injectable testosterone preparations require long half-lives to be given as depot, which results in wide fluctuations in plasma testosterone concentrations.

Transdermal preparations are most frequently used.

Gels reduce localised skin side-effects compared to traditional testosterone patches; however, the patient has to ensure skin is not touched by others (e.g. partner, children).

Table 7 – Comparison of different administration routes for TRT

Route	Example
Oral	e.g. testosterone undecanoate, 40–120mg (PO) daily
Intramuscular	e.g. testosterone undecanoate, 1g (IM) every 12 weeks
Transdermal	Testogel® 40.5mg/2.5g, apply 40.5mg daily

MALE INFERTILITY

MALE REPRODUCTIVE PHYSIOLOGY

The hypothalamic–pituitary–gonadal axis is shown in Figure 3.

GnRH from the hypothalamus causes pulsatile release of FSH/LH from the anterior pituitary gland which in turn acts on the testis.

LH makes Leydig cells produce testosterone, whilst FSH stimulates inhibin and sperm production.

In the serum, testosterone is either free (2%), or bound to albumin (38%), or bound to SHBG (60%).

In androgen-responsive tissues, 5α-reductase converts testosterone to its more potent form DHT.

Testosterone is the primary negative feedback hormone to further pituitary release of LH.

Figure 3 – Hypothalamo–pituitary–gonadal axis

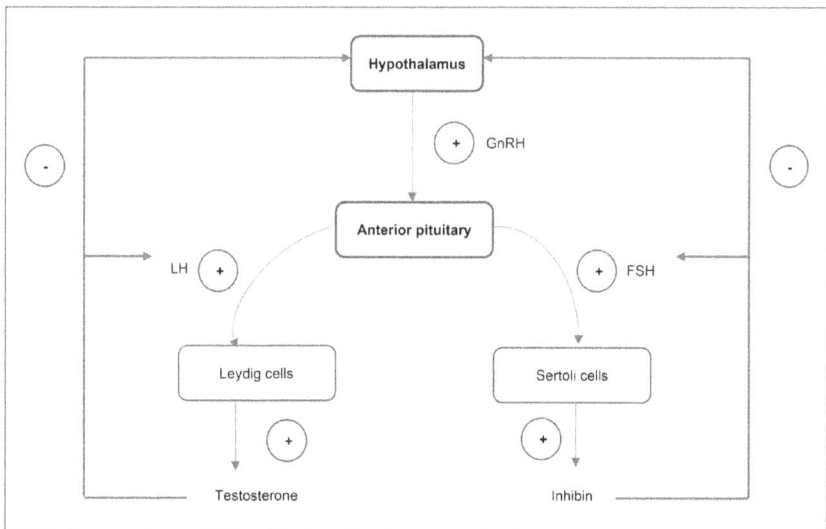

SPERMATOGENESIS

Seminiferous tubules are lined with Sertoli cells, which provide nutrients to germ cells.

Type-A spermatogonia are stem cells – they can self-renew (remaining as type A) or differentiate to sperm (type B).

Primordial germ cells

(x1 type-B spermatogonium) -> mitosis -> primary spermatocytes (x2 diploid)

(first meiotic division) -> secondary spermatocytes (46 chromosomes) (x4)

(second meiotic division) -> spermatids (23 chromosomes) (x8)

(spermiogenesis) -> spermatozoa (entire process 72 days)

(i.e. one type-B spermatogonium will yield 8 spermatozoa.)

These are stored and matured in the epididymis; however, they spend most of their life in the testis.

Sperm motility increases during epididymal transit, due to increased capacity for glycolysis.

Sperm is viable for ≤ 5 days in the female.

DEFINITIONS

Infertility defined as inability to achieve pregnancy within 12 months of regular unprotected sex:

- *Primary*, refers to couple that have never had a child
- *Secondary*, couples who have been able to achieve pregnancy at least once.

Azoospermia – absent sperm in ejaculate.

Oligospermia – abnormality of low sperm numbers (< 15 x 106/mL).

Asthenospermia – abnormality of motility (< 40% motile), progressive motility < 32%.

Teratozoospermia – abnormality of morphology (< 4% normal forms).

Globozoospermia – sperm lack acrosomal caps (rendered spherical), natural conception is not possible.

Necrospermia – high percentage of dead/immotile sperm (test with vitality staining).

OAT syndrome refers to combined defects of sperm motility, morphology and density (oligoasthenoteratospermia) can be caused by varicocele, cryptorchidism, heat.

EPIDEMIOLOGY

Generally ≤ 85% of people will conceive within 12 months if they have frequent unprotected sex.

Around 1 in 7 couples may have difficulty conceiving in the UK.

1/3 of infertility cases are caused by male reproductive issues, 1/3 by female reproductive issues, and 1/3 by both male and female (i.e. a male factor infertility is present in ≤ 50% of cases).

Azoospermia is present in 1% of male population.

1 in 3 men with impaired sperm parameters have no clear underlying cause to account for this.

Rising prevalence of male factor infertility is thought to be due to advancing average paternal age.

SEMEN CHARACTERISTICS

Semen analysis is a key test in the evaluation of the infertile male. [13]

Recommended that patient abstains from ejaculation for 2–5 days prior to producing sample.

Sample should be provided in clean container ideally directly in laboratory, or delivered within 1 hour of production whilst kept warm in transit, without use of condoms or spermicide.

If sample result is normal, as per WHO criteria, a single test is sufficient.

Any repeat sample should be delivered ≥ 3 months from last (full spermatogenesis cycle).

Coitus interruptus sample not recommended as acidic vaginal secretions may contaminate this.

The majority of the ejaculate volume is derived from the seminal vesicles (~70%).

NICE (last updated 2017) continues to use WHO fifth edition (2010) thresholds for semen parameters; however, WHO sixth edition (2021) has since been published, with slight modifications (Table 8).

Table 8 – WHO fifth (2010) and sixth (2021) editions semen analysis parameters [14]

Parameter	Lower Limit (2010)	Lower Limit (2021)
Semen volume (mL)	1.5	1.4
Total sperm count (106)	39	39
Sperm concentration (106/mL)	15	16
Progressive motility (PR %)	32	30
Vitality (live spermatozoa %)	58	54
Sperm morphology (normal forms %)	4	4
pH	> 7.2	≥ 7.2

The *mixed agglutination reaction* test is used to detect anti-sperm antibodies, which can be useful in evaluating immunological infertility.

Distribution of male infertility by semen analysis:

- Multiple abnormalities (49%)
- Normal (14%)
- Azoospermia (14%)
- Single abnormality: low volume (7%), asthenospermia (6%), oligospermia (4%).

Further evaluation of male infertility is directed towards the predominant semen analysis finding.

VIVA   If an infertility station arises in your FRCS (Urol) viva, you will almost certainly be given a semen analysis result to interpret and discuss. I therefore recommend you practise interpreting these via your own method that allows you to systematically work through any semen analysis result, permitting you not only to name the type of semen abnormality but also potential causes of that abnormality.

AETIOLOGY

There are many potential causes of male factor infertility:

- *Idiopathic* – seen in ≤ 33% of cases
- *Congenital*, such as anorchia, cryptorchidism, genetic (e.g. Klinefelter, Kartagener, CF)
- *Trauma*
- *Testicular torsion*
- *Hormonal*, such as prolactinoma, steroid abuse, CAH, low FSH/LH/ testosterone
- *Systemic*, such as liver/renal failure
- *Varicocele*
- *Previous chemotherapy*
- *Infective*, such as STI, mumps orchitis
- Recreational drugs, such as anabolic steroids and marijuana.

The top 3 male factors are varicocele, idiopathic and obstructive (endocrine only accounts for ~2%).

Figure 4 – Male factor infertility

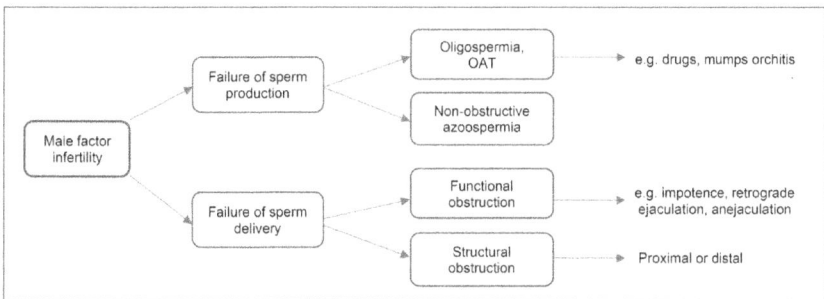

DIAGNOSTIC EVALUATION

Patient History

A thorough history, preferably with female partner present, should be undertaken in a dedicated fertility clinic with fertility nurse specialist present, evaluating:

- Duration of infertility (> 12 months), frequency and timing of intercourse
- Details of previous conceptions/births (i.e. primary vs. secondary)
- Erectile and ejaculatory function
- Use of vaginal lubricants (as these can be spermicidal)
- Sexual development history
- Detailed past medical and drug history to screen for risk factors as listed above.

Patient Examination

Examine the consenting patient in the presence of chaperone.

Commence by general inspection – recording BMI, signs of development of secondary sexual characteristics/virilisation pattern.

Proceed then to focused urological examination to evaluate:

- Testes for size, consistency and number
- Presence of varicocele
- Whether both vas deferens are palpable in the scrotum
- Epididymis for signs of blockage/granuloma.

The partner should undergo full assessment in a dedicated gynaecological clinic for infertility.

A longitudinal axis < 4.6cm measured with calliper orchidometer is associated with potential impairment in spermatogenesis.

INVESTIGATIONS

Baseline

Request blood tests for LH, FSH and testosterone (as well as viral screen e.g. hepatitis B and C, HIV).

Interpretations of the results are shown in Table 9.

Table 9 – Diagnostic interpretation of combined FSH, LH and testosterone results

FSH	LH	Testosterone	Potential Cause
High	Normal	Normal	Seminiferous tubule damage
Normal	Normal	Normal	Genital tract obstruction
High	High	Normal	Testicular failure
Low	Low	Low	Hypogonadotropism

A raised FSH suggests testes are not working; reduced FSH suggests intracranial pathology; normal FSH may suggest underlying obstructive cause.

Two separate semen analyses are recommended to confirm an abnormal result.

Pasqualini syndrome features an isolated deficiency in LH.

Imaging

Scrotal US may be helpful to evaluate:

- Testicular volume
- Testicular anatomy, dysgenesis, tumours
- Indirect signs of obstruction (rete testis dilatation, absent vas deferens)
- Underlying varicocele.

TRUS can be helpful to assess for ejaculatory duct cysts/calculi causing obstruction.

Vasography

A vasogram involves puncture of vas deferens within scrotum and injection of contrast, which if normal should flow freely through vas into bladder.

Should be done ideally at time of planned reconstructive surgery (vas damage may occur that might complicate future surgery).

TESTICULAR BIOPSY

Performed in azoospermia to differentiate between obstructive and non-obstructive causes.

Sperm can be retrieved simultaneously for use in assisted conception, as long as it is sufficiently mature on the *Johnsen score* (≥ 8, range 1–10).

Biopsy is rarely performed in isolation.

Biopsy is not routinely indicated in oligospermia as it does not affect treatment options.

Biopsy is not routinely indicated in azoospermia if normal testes volume and gonadotrophins and CBAVD – patient needs counselling for cystic fibrosis screening followed by TESE.

The *Johnsen score count* is used to classify spermatogenesis on a testicular biopsy (Table 10).

Table 10 – Johnsen score used as histological grading system for testicular biopsy

Score	Description
1	No cells, tubular fibrosis
2	Sertoli cells only
3	Spermatogonia
4	< 10 spermatocytes
5	No spermatozoa, many spermatocytes
6	No spermatozoa, but < 10 spermatids
7	No spermatozoa, but many spermatids
8	< 10 spermatozoa
9	Many spermatozoa – disorganised epithelium
10	Complete spermatogenesis

OLIGOSPERMIA

Defined as sperm concentration < 16 x 106/mL of ejaculate:

- If < 10 x 106, consider karyotyping
- If < 5 x 106, consider Y-microdeletion test.

Common causes include varicocele, androgen deficiency and idiopathic.

In addition to a full detailed infertility patient history, the following tests should be considered:

- Hormone profile (raised FSH may suggest seminiferous tubular failure)
- Serum prolactin (hyperprolactinaemia may adversely affect spermatogenesis)
- US scrotum to evaluate for varicocele.

Isolated FSH elevation indicates failure of spermatogenesis rather than endocrine abnormality.

Treatment mainly involves addressing underlying cause (if found) or assisted conception.

AZOOSPERMIA

Defined as absence of sperm within the ejaculate; can be obstructive (40%) or non-obstructive (60%).

The following are obstructive causes of azoospermia:

- Vas deferens, e.g. CBAVD (associated with CF), vasectomy, previous scrotal/hernia surgery
- Epididymal, such as post-infective or post-surgery
- Ejaculatory duct (e.g. anejaculation in SCI).

Obstructive causes are more common in patients with normal testes and hormone profile, with a semen analysis suggesting azoospermia.

The following are non-obstructive causes:

- Hormonal, such as hypogonadotropism
- Abnormalities of spermatogenesis, such as trauma/torsion, mumps, Klinefelter's.

Azoospermia Investigations

Hormone profile blood tests (LH/FSH/testosterone) should all return normal.

Azoospermic semen sample should be repeated to confirm finding.

TRUS can assess vas and/or ejaculatory duct obstruction, consider vasogram and/or testicular biopsy.

Chromosomal analyses are not routinely recommended; consider if Klinefelter's is suspected (azoospermia, small testes, low FSH/LH/ testosterone, gynaecomastia).

Table 11 – Test result profile for different aetiological causes of azoospermia

	Distal Obstruction	Proximal Obstruction	Retrograde Ejaculation	Anejaculation (e.g. SCI)
FSH	normal	normal	normal	normal
Testes Volume	normal	normal	normal	normal
Semen Volume	normal	low	low/none	none
Sperm Count	azoospermia	azoospermia	azoospermia	azoospermia
Fructose/pH	normal	low, acidic	normal	n/a
Post-ejaculate Urinanalysis	normal	normal	> 10 sperm/ HPF	n/a

Azoospermia Management

The management plan will depend on the underlying cause that has been identified (e.g. hormonal replacement, reconstructive surgery or assisted conception).

CBAVD will require assisted conception techniques.

If a tubular obstructive cause is identified then surgical excision and anastomosis can be performed (microsurgical vaso-vasostomy or tubulovasostomy).

Ejaculatory duct obstruction is an uncommon cause of obstructive azoospermia, accounting for < 5% of male infertility cases due to obstructive causes.

May arise congenitally (Mullerian or Wolffian duct cysts) or acquired (calculus).

Findings may include azoo-/oligospermia with low semen fructose/volume/pH; TRUS evaluation may reveal dilated seminal vesicles.

Ejaculatory duct obstruction is treated by TURED – seminal vesicles are filled with methylene blue (via trans-rectal needle), surgeon then resects the verumontanum until a blue flush is seen.

Patency rates ≤ 90%, fertility ≤ 40%.

Y-MICRODELETIONS

Microdeletions of Y-chromosome are the second most frequent genetic cause of spermatogenic failure in infertile men, after Klinefelter's syndrome.

Patients usually phenotypically normal, with the only abnormality being a defect in spermatogenesis.

The defect occurs in one of three non-overlapping regions of the long arm of Y-chromosome.

These microdeletions are referred to as:

- AZFa (proximal), Sertoli only (cannot father children)
- AZFb (middle), maturation arrest (cannot father children)
- AZFc (distal), severe oligospermia (50% success rate with micro-TESE; however, all male offspring will be infertile).

Y-microdeletions usually result in non-obstructive azoospermia or severe oligospermia.

Men with AZFa or AZFb will not have sperm within testicle and therefore retrieval is not indicated, whilst there is a small chance (10%) of finding sperm in AZFc.

All male offspring of men with microdeletions will inherit the same deletion.

AZFa/AZFb have to be advised regarding sperm donation or adoption.

VARICOCELE AND MALE INFERTILITY

Varicocele is present in ~15% of normal male population, in 25% of men with abnormal semen parameters and in ≤ 40% of men presenting with infertility.

The exact association between reduced male fertility and varicocele is unknown, and the subject of varicocele repair in context of treating infertility has been long debated.

Surgical varicocelectomy improves semen parameters in those men whose parameters are abnormal.

No benefit in pregnancy rates consistently found by correcting varicocele if semen parameters normal.

EAU 2024 recommends for infertile men:

- Not to treat varicocele if semen parameters are normal
- Treat varicocele if this is clinically apparent and semen parameters are abnormal and otherwise unexplained infertility, where female partner has good ovarian reserve.

Please see more in "Varicocele" section.

MALE ASSISTED CONCEPTION

There are many assisted conception techniques, as listed in Table 12.

Table 12 – Techniques of assisted conception and their abbreviations

Technique	Abbreviation
Intra-uterine insemination	IUI
In-vitro fertilisation	IVF
Intra-cytoplasmic sperm injection	ICSI
Microsurgical epididymal sperm aspiration	MESA
Percutaneous sperm aspiration	PESA
Testicular sperm extraction	TESE
Micro testicular sperm extraction	mTESE
Testicular sperm aspiration	TESA

INTRA-UTERINE INSEMINATION

IUI is used to bypass cervical mucus by placing sperm directly into uterus.

Sperm must be processed to remove bacteria and prostaglandins, which are irritants to the uterus, often done concomitantly with ovarian hyperstimulation to improve pregnancy rates.

Indications for IUI include:

- Deposition abnormality (e.g. uncorrected hypospadias)
- Severe dyspareunia
- Severe psychosexual abnormalities or physical disabilities.

Outcomes include pregnancy rates $\leq$ 30% for 4 cycles and multiple gestation in up to 30%.

Success rates for IUI are generally around a third of that for IVF, but it costs a quarter of the price.

IVF AND ICSI

Initial ovarian hyperstimulation with clomiphene is then followed by transvaginal egg harvest.

Sperm fertilisation occurs in culture medium in a laboratory; 2–5 days of growth; 1–2 fertilised eggs are then placed into the uterus.

Success rates of IVF decline with age (32% for women < 35 years, 5% for women aged 43 years).

NICE has set out eligibility criteria for IVF on the NHS:

- $\leq$ 3 cycles for women < 40 years who have not conceived after 2 years of regular sex
- 1 cycle for women aged 40–42 years who have not conceived after 2 years of regular sex, provided they have not had a previous IVF cycle.

ICSI is similar to IVF in the steps followed before and after insemination, differing only in the actual laboratory process utilised to fertilise the egg.

A single sperm cell is injected directly into the cytoplasm of an egg.

ICSI may be considered in the following circumstances:

- Severe problem with sperm quality (e.g. high percentage of abnormal shapes or poor motility)
- When previous IVF failed to fertilise any eggs
- Sperm retrieved surgically (e.g. TESE or PESA).

SPERM-RETRIEVAL TECHNIQUES

Sperm-retrieval techniques are indicated when surgical reconstruction is not possible.

MESA and PESA have equivalent pregnancy rates.

TESE conventionally involves single/multiple testicular biopsies to retrieve seminiferous tubules, which are then dissected to retrieve mature sperm to use for assisted conception.

mTESE utilises high magnification of seminiferous tubules to target the best ones for extraction, which can then be frozen for future ICSI or sperm harvested for same day ICSI cycle.

PEYRONIE'S DISEASE

Peyronie's disease is an acquired condition characterised by deformity of the penile shaft secondary to the formation of a fibrous scar on the tunica albuginea.

Congenital penile curvature is rare, results from disproportionate development of tunica albuginea of the corporal bodies, not associated with urethral malformation, deviation usually ventral.

Patients usually present after onset of puberty.

EPIDEMIOLOGY

Peyronie's disease is likely under-reported – estimated prevalence ≤ 10%.

Typical age of onset is 50–60 years.

≤ 50% of patients with Peyronie's disease have depression, ~20% have Dupuytren's contracture.

AETIOLOGY

The pathophysiology of Peyronie's disease is not fully understood.

It is considered to be a wound-healing disorder which occurs after penile trauma in predisposed men, due to microvascular injury and bleeding into tunica resulting in inflammation and fibrosis.

Natural progression of Peyronie's disease:

- 40% progress within 1 year
- 14% resolve spontaneously
- 50% approximately experience stabilisation.

The plaques have extensive connective tissue with random collagen orientation (most common dorsally) – *transforming growth factor beta* (TGF-β1) is typically over-expressed.

Two phases of the disease can be distinguished: *active/inflammatory* and *stable/fibrotic*.

Peyronie's disease often occurs alongside ED, due to altered haemodynamics of cavernosal blood flow.

Active Phase

The acute inflammatory phase lasts ≤ 6 months.

Patient may experience pain in flaccid and/or erect state, progressive curvature will start to develop possibly along with a palpable plaque the patient can feel.

Stable Phase

The chronic fibrotic phase lasts subsequently ≤ 12 months.

Penile pain disappears in most patients (≤ 90%) and the curvature should stop getting worse; however, spontaneous improvement is unusual (~14%).

Surgical treatment should be deferred until after the stable phase is established.

RISK FACTORS

The most commonly associated comorbidities with Peyronie's disease are:

- Diabetes
- Smoking and excessive alcohol
- Hypertension, IHD, lipid abnormalities
- Dupuytren's contracture
- Ledderhose's disease (plantar-fascial contracture)
- Previous penile trauma.

DIAGNOSTIC EVALUATION

History

History and examination are key to diagnosing Peyronie's disease.

Key factors to be established in the patient history include:

- Duration and progression of symptoms
- Presence of pain (active vs. stable disease)
- Presence of ED and any medications already used to help with this
- Degree of curvature (patient may have photographic evidence)
- Risk factors and associated comorbidities
- Impact of the condition on patient's sex life and wellbeing.

Ask patient to complete validated questionnaire such as IIEF-5 (although this has not been formally validated for Peyronie's disease).

There is an alternative *Peyronie's disease questionnaire* (PDQ).

Examination

The examination of the patient should be conducted in the presence of a chaperone.

Examination of external genitalia should be performed for palpable plaque (more common on dorsal aspect) – plaque size does not correlate with degree of curvature.

Examine hands and feet for evidence of Dupuytren's contracture or Ledderhose scarring.

Objective evaluation of penile curvature is important to record via (artificially induced) erection:

- Degree of curvature
- Flaccid and erect penile length (important if surgery is planned).

US not recommended to measure plaque; Doppler may only be relevant for vascular parameters.

Medical photography with signed consent is preferable: lateral, frontal and views from above.

If the deviation is ventral, particularly in a younger patient, this should raise suspicion they may have congenital curvature abnormality.

MANAGEMENT

CONSERVATIVE

Non-operative management is advocated for early Peyronie's disease in the active phase.

Peyronie's disease does not mandate treatment if patient is not troubled by condition; common symptoms that impact QOL include ED and inability to penetrate.

A small proportion of cases (14%) will resolve spontaneously, and half will not progress.

MEDICAL

There are many proposed medical options available to treat Peyronie's disease; however, many have not undergone rigorous evaluation in controlled clinical trials.

Many agents rely on anecdotal evidence to support their usage, which is often contradictory.

Overall oral therapies have proved disappointing.

PDE5-inhibitors

PDE5i were thought to reduce collagen deposition and increase apoptosis by inhibiting TGF-β.

EAU 2024 supports their use for concomitant ED and/or to optimise penetration.

ESWL

The therapeutic mechanism of action of ESWL in treating Peyronie's disease is unclear.

ESWL may work by damaging/remodelling the plaque or by increasing its vascularity.

ESWL may help to reduce pain and EAU 2024 supports its use as analgesic; however, it has not been shown to be beneficial for treating curvature.

Intra-lesional Treatment

Injection of pharmacologically active agent directly into penile plaque allows localised delivery which provides higher concentrations of the drug inside the plaque.

Injecting IFN-α2b has been shown to improve deformity and pain and is supported by EAU 2024.

Intra-lesional injection of steroids, hyaluronic acid or botulinum toxin is not recommended.

Clostridium Collagenase

Clostridium collagenase (marketed as Xiapex®) as intra-lesional injection is the only drug approved for the treatment of Peyronie's disease by the FDA and EMA.

It has since been officially withdrawn in 2019 from the European market.

Xiapex® is not available on the NHS in the UK, and may only be administered as a private treatment.

Clostridium collagenase is an enzyme that attacks collagen (primary component of Peyronie's plaque).

Injections may cause penile pain, bruising and swelling as most common side-effects.

There is no consensus on number of injections/cycles that should be given; however, patient is encouraged in between injections to perform penis mechanical modelling.

Clostridium collagenase shown to be effective (15–20° improvement) with good safety profile.

Penile Traction Devices

Traction and/or vacuum devices have been shown to beneficial in the pre- and post-operative Peyronie's disease setting, preferably in conjunction with other treatments.

Can increase/preserve penile length, encourages tissue modelling, must be used $\geq$ 3 hours/day.

EAU 2024 supports use of traction devices as part of multi-modal therapy.

POTABA, Vitamin E, Tamoxifen

EAU 2024 does not recommend using POTABA, vitamin E or tamoxifen.

Potassium para-aminobenzoate (POTABA) is a drug used to treat disorders associated with formation of excess fibrous tissue in the body (e.g. Peyronie's disease, scleroderma).

POTABA works by increasing the uptake of oxygen into the tissue. [15]

Tamoxifen is an oestrogen receptor antagonist that modulates TGFβ-1 secretion by fibroblasts, believed to be more effective in the acute inflammatory phase.

Vitamin E works by inactivating free radicals that saturate NO, thereby keeping active NO levels high to promote wound healing and offer anti-inflammatory action. [16]

SURGICAL

Surgery is indicated in fit patients with stable Peyronie's disease (≥ 3 months) with the aim of correcting penile curvature and allowing penetrative intercourse.

Prior to surgical intervention the following should be recorded:

- Degree of curvature
- Complex deformities (e.g. hourglass or hinge)
- Stretched and erect penile lengths
- Presence of ED
- Presence of foreskin (which may need removing at time of surgery).

The 3 main types of reconstruction to be considered for Peyronie's disease are:

- *Convex-shortening* (Nesbit/Yachia/plication)
- *Concave-lengthening* (plaque incision and grafting)
- Prosthesis insertion with or without straightening techniques.

Tunical Shortening Surgery

Tunical shortening procedures involve plication techniques (e.g. Nesbit) – also called corporoplasty.

Plication surgery is recommended in mild/moderate Peyronie's disease (< 60°) with good erections.

Nesbit procedure involves:

- De-gloving penis via circumglanular incision
- Induction of artificial erection to reveal site of maximal deformity
- Elliptical excision of tunica albuginea opposite to the point of maximum curvature (1mm for every 10° curve), close defect with sutures
- Patients commonly experience penile shortening.

Success rates > 80%, recurrence of curvature is uncommon and ED as a complication is rare (1%).

Yachia procedure is a less common alternative – involves multiple longitudinal incisions in tunica which are closed horizontally.

Tunical Lengthening Surgery

Tunical lengthening procedures involve excision/incision of plaque with defect filled by a graft.

Generally recommended in patients with severe curvature (> 60°) and/or complex deformities but with good erectile function (with or without reliance on PDE5i drugs).

Incision undertaken in the short (concave) side to increase this side's length, with the aim of relaxing the tunica completely.

Lue procedure involves plaque incision with insertion of venous patch to lengthen affected side:

- Saphenous vein is the most common autograft (followed by dorsal penile vein)
- Alternative graft materials include autograft (tunica vaginalis), allograft (cadaveric pericardium), xenograft (e.g. porcine small intestine, bovine pericardium).

Lue procedure has higher risk of ED (≤ 25%), much lower of penile shortening (≤ 20%).

Penile Implants

Peyronie's disease associated with refractory ED should be treated with penile prosthesis implantation.

Inflatable prostheses are generally preferable to patients over malleable devices.

The risk of urethral injury (5%) during prosthesis insertion is greater for Peyronie's disease patients as opposed to patients having a prosthesis for ED only.

Deformities ≤ 30° after implant insertion are likely to resolve once pump is used for 6 months.

Severe hourglass deformity with good erectile function may require grafting and penile prosthesis.

Peyronie's Disease Surgery Algorithm

Figure 5 – PD surgery algorithm

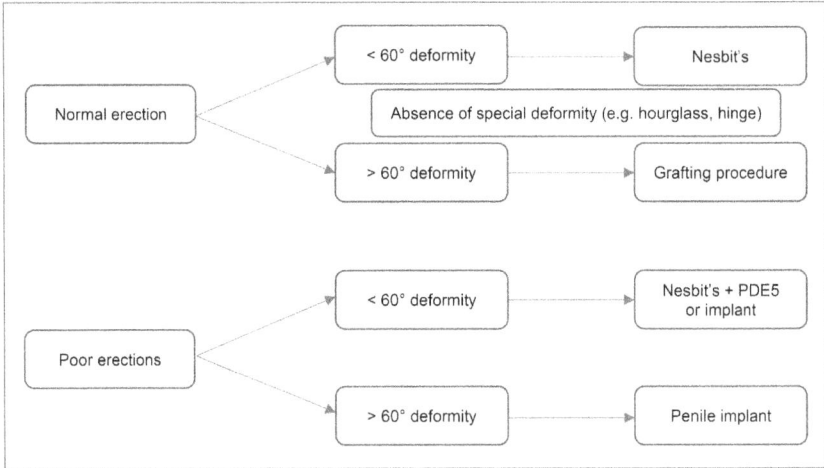

LUTS DIAGNOSTIC EVALUATION

LUTS should be broadly divided into storage and voiding symptoms.

LUTS are strongly associated with ageing.

They were traditionally related to BOO due to BPE; however, LUTS are often related to the prostate, such as bladder dysfunction (e.g. DO, OAB) or prostatic inflammation.

HISTORY

A thorough medical and surgical history must be taken from men with LUTS.

Prior to attending the clinic the patient should be requested to complete a 3-day bladder diary.

The key aspects in the history include:

- Description of symptoms to determine whether these are voiding or storage predominant
- Associated red-flag symptoms
- Associated UTI
- Relevant comorbidities/urological history
- Current medication
- Lifestyle habits
- Impact on QOL and what is patient's goal.

Nocturia is the hardest symptom to fix by means of bladder outflow surgery.

A validated symptom score questionnaire should be used to evaluate male LUTS, which also allows for disease monitoring or reassessment after treatment.

The IPSS questionnaire features (Table 13):

- 7 symptom questions
- 1 QOL question
- Does not include incontinence
- Score ranges from 0–35: *asymptomatic* (0), *mild* (1–7), *moderate* (8–19) and severe (20–35).

An increase > 4 points on the IPSS is related to a subjective worsening of bother of urinary symptoms.

Alternatives include the *Danish Prostate Symptom Score* and *AUA Symptom Score*.

Table 13 – IPSS questionnaire and additional quality of life question

In the Past Month:	Not at All	Less than 1/5 Times	Less than ½ the Time	About ½ the Time	More than ½ the Time	Almost Always
1. Incomplete Emptying How often have you had a sensation of not emptying your bladder completely after you finish urinating?	0	1	2	3	4	5
2. Frequency How often have you had to urinate again less than two hours after you finished urinating?	0	1	2	3	4	5
3. Intermittency How often have you found you stopped and started again several times when you urinated?	0	1	2	3	4	5
4. Urgency How difficult have you found it to postpone going to pass urine?	0	1	2	3	4	5
5. Weak Stream How often have you had a weak urinary stream?	0	1	2	3	4	5
6. Straining How often have you had to push or strain to begin urination?	0	1	2	3	4	5

	None	Once	Twice	3x	4x	≥ 5x
7. Nocturia How many times did you most typically get up to urinate from bedtime until waking up in morning?	0	1	2	3	4	5

Quality of Life Question	Delighted	Pleased	Mostly Satisfied	Mixed	Mostly Dissatisfied	Unhappy	Terrible
If you were to live the rest of your life with your urinary symptoms as they are now, how would you feel?	0	1	2	3	4	5	6

VIVA | I recommend you learn the entire IPSS questionnaire including the final score categories thoroughly for the FRCS (Urol), as you will be expected to know this without prompting.

EXAMINATION

Complete a thorough patient examination with consent, in the presence of a chaperone.

The key aspects of patient examination include:

- Abdomen for palpable bladder, masses, scars
- External genitalia for phimosis or meatal pathology
- DRE for prostate size, contour or tenderness
- Evaluation for stigmata of renal and/or neurological disease.

Complete examination with urine dipstick +/- MSU for culture, and PVR.

INVESTIGATIONS

BASELINE/BEDSIDE TESTS

The appropriate tests will be determined by the patient history and examination, as well as presence of UTI and/or red-flag symptoms.

An accurately completed FVC or bladder diary should be undertaken in the assessment of male LUTS (EAU 2024); patients should be counselled on how to complete one over minimum 3-day period.

FVC details the volume and time of each void by the patient.

Bladder diary includes additional information such as fluid intake, relevant symptoms such as urgency, use of pads and incontinence episodes.

Urinalysis should be completed (EAU 2024).

Blood tests should be considered including:

- UE, if renal impairment is suspected, or hydronephrosis noted, or prior to LUTS surgery
- PSA, if DRE abnormal, strong family history of PCa, patient request
- FBC and HBA1c if history of rUTI.

PSA is a stronger predictor of prostate growth than prostate volume is, and can also be used as a predictor for risk of AUR and need for BOO-related surgery.

IMAGING

PVR must be recorded in the evaluation of male LUTS (EAU 2024).

PVR can be assessed via formal trans-abdominal US, bedside bladder scan or catheterisation.

A high PVR does not necessarily imply patient has BOO, as it may arise due to poor detrusor function; however, it can be used as monitoring tool to predict risk of progression to AUR event.

Consider upper-tract imaging via US or CT if:

- History of red-flag symptoms
- Presence of UTI or sterile pyuria
- Previous urolithiasis.

Imaging of the prostate is recommended when considering surgical treatment (EAU 2024).

FLEXIBLE CYSTOSCOPY

Flexible cystoscopy should not be used as a routine initial test to evaluate male LUTS unless:

- History of visible haematuria or rUTI
- Profound symptoms or pain
- Previous urethral stricture or bladder cancer.

Perform flexible cystoscopy if considering UroLift to evaluate for presence of median lobe.

There is no strong correlation between flexible cystoscopy and UDS findings.

UROFLOWMETRY

Uroflowmetry should be used for initial assessment of male LUTS and prior to invasive treatment, and can also be used to monitor/evaluate treatment outcomes.

A flow-rate test should be evaluated with a voided volume > 150mL.

Normal age-specific flow rates (Qmax) for men are:

- < 40 years   = > 21mL/s
- 40–60 years   = > 18mL/s
- > 60 years   = > 13mL/s.

A reduced Qmax is usually evidence of BOO.

90% of men with Qmax < 10mL/s will have UDS evidence of obstruction, the remaining 10% will have evidence of reduced detrusor contractility.

75% of men with Qmax > 15mL/s will not have BOO, the remaining 25% who are obstructed maintain their flow by increasing detrusor contraction intensity.

As an approximate guide to uroflowmetry interpretation:

- Qmax < 10mL/s   = 90% chance of obstruction
- Qmax 10–15mL/s   = 60% chance of obstruction
- Qmax > 15mL/s   = 10% chance of obstruction.

Flow-rate meters are covered in Chapter 6, "Urological Imaging & Principles of Urological Technology".

URODYNAMICS

Routine UDS should not be requested unless (EAU 2024):

- Previously unsuccessful invasive LUTS treatment/surgery
- Co-existing neurological disease
- Men who cannot void > 150mL
- Considering surgery in men with predominantly voiding LUTS and PVR > 300mL
- Considering surgery in men with predominantly voiding LUTS and age > 80 years or < 50 years.

Recall the relevant ICS nomogram based on UDS findings as per Figure 6.

Figure 6 – ICS nomogram based on UDS findings

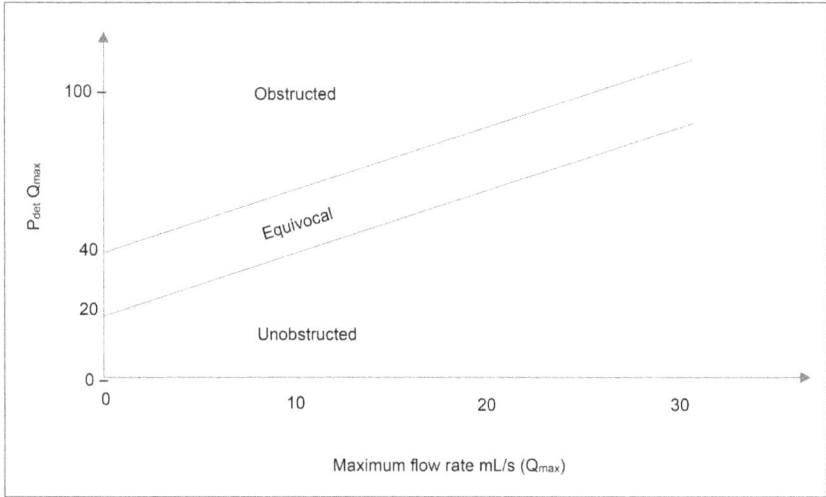

Bladder Outlet Obstruction Index (Abrams–Griffiths number) = (PdetQmax) – (2Qmax)

- *unobstructed < 20, equivocal 20–40, obstructed > 40*

TREATMENT OF BPH

WATCHFUL WAITING

Many men with LUTS are not sufficiently troubled by their symptoms to need or want treatment.

Patient should be counselled about lifestyle modifications:

- Reduction of caffeinated beverages and alcohol
- Avoid drinking before bedtime
- Bladder retraining techniques.

WW is a viable option for such men, as few progress to AUR and related complications, even when their IPSS score is severe.

Symptoms are likely to deteriorate with age; however, the overall extent of this is low.

Factors that can predict disease progression include:

- Failure to respond to medical therapy or symptom deterioration whilst on treatment
- Increasing PVR
- Presence of inflammation on TRUS biopsies
- PSA ≥ 1.4ng/mL
- Previous AUR.

Risk factors for AUR are shown in Table 14.

Table 14 – Risk factors for developing AUR in male patients with LUTS

Risk Factor	AUR Relative Risk
IPSS > 7	3.2
Qmax < 12mL/s	3.9
Prostate vol. > 30mL	3.0
PSA > 1.4	2.0
Age > 70 years vs. 40–49 years	10–11
Unspecified volume of PVR	

KEY PAPER | Olmsted County Study (1999) [17]

- Longitudinal study, 6-year follow-up of 2,115 men with LUTS.
- Evaluating risk of AUR and need for BOO surgery.
- Demonstrated that BPH is age dependent and progressive, IPSS rises by 0.18 points/year, Q_{max} decreases 2%/year and risk of AUR increases with age.
- Identified risk factors for BPH progression and requirement of surgical treatment (Table 14).

MEDICAL THERAPY

α-1 ADRENORECEPTOR ANTAGONISTS

Inhibit NA effect on prostatic smooth muscle by blocking α-1 adrenoreceptors, thereby reducing tone.

α-1 blockers have little effect on UDS-determined BOO.

There are two broad sub-types of α-adrenoreceptor:

- α-1 (with sub-types α-1a, α-1b and α-1L)
- α-2.

The α-1 blockers are classified by their adrenoreceptor selectivity and elimination half-life (Table 15).

Table 15 – The different classifications of α-1 blockers

Selectivity	α-1 Blocker
Non-selective	Phenoxybenzamine
α-1	Prazosin, alfuzosin
Long acting α-1	Terazosin, doxazosin
Sub-type selective α-1a (more than α-1b)	Tamsulosin

Efficacy

All α-1 blockers appear to have comparable clinical efficacies in their appropriate doses – benefits can be noted within hours/days; however, full effect takes several weeks.

α-1 blockers reduce IPSS by approximately 30–40% and increase Qmax by ~25%.

Benefit is similar across all age groups.

NICE recommends α-1 blockers to treat men with moderate-to-severe LUTS with planned review after 6 weeks and then at least yearly.

Side-effects

α-1 adrenoreceptors located outside the prostate (e.g. blood vessels, CNS) mediate for the drug-specific side-effects.

The most common side-effects of α-1 blockers include:

- Asthenia (weakness)
- Dizziness and postural hypotension
- Retrograde ejaculation
- Floppy iris syndrome during cataract surgery (i.e. inform ophthalmologist); risk of posterior capsule rupture may not disappear even if medication is stopped.

5α-REDUCTASE INHIBITORS

5ARIs work on the static component of BPE, reducing prostatic volume ≤ 25% after 6–12 months.

Testosterone, via the enzyme 5α-reductase, is converted to DHT which has more potent androgenic effects on the prostate. 5ARIs work by competitive inhibition of 5α-reductase.

There are 2 isoforms of the 5α-reductase enzyme:

- *Type 1* – minor expression in prostate (mainly in skin and liver)
- *Type 2* – predominant expression and activity in the prostate.

Two 5ARIs are in clinical use – dutasteride (inhibits type 1 and 2) and finasteride (inhibits type 2 only):

- Serum reduction of DHT with dutasteride (95%) and finasteride (70%)
- Prostate DHT reduction similar for both around 90%
- Approximately halving the patient's PSA reading within 12 months.

Clinical efficacy of dutasteride and finasteride are comparable.

Patients must be counselled regarding the delayed symptomatic improvement with 5ARIs.

NICE recommends 5ARIs be offered to treat LUTS in any of the following circumstances:

- Prostate estimated > 30g in size
- PSA > 1.4ng/mL
- High risk of progression (e.g. older age, previous AUR).

EAU 2024 recommends 5ARIs in men who have moderate-to-severe LUTS and an increased risk of disease progression.

Efficacy

5ARIs are less effective when used as monotherapy compared to α-1 blockers; however, they help reduce disease progression.

5ARIs (not α-1 blockers) reduce long-term risk of AUR (57%) or BOO surgery (55%) at 4 years.

After 2–4 years of 5ARI treatment:

- IPSS improvement of 15–30%
- Decrease prostate volume ≤ 25%
- Increase Qmax by ≤ 2mL/s.

5ARIs may reduce bleeding during TURP surgery due to effects on prostatic revascularisation (suppression of VEGF).

Side-effects

Side-effects are generally mild and related to problems with sexual function, such as ED, reduced libido, gynaecomastia (1–2%) and ejaculation disorders.

Counsel the patient regarding 5ARIs and PCa – lower prevalence of PCa with finasteride; however, with a higher incidence of high-grade tumours (PCPT Trial).

KEY PAPER | PLESS Study (1998) [18]

- PLESS (Proscar Long-term Efficacy and Safety Study) where Proscar is finasteride.
- Multi-centre, randomised, placebo-controlled trial of 3,000+ men with BPH over 4 years.
- Randomised to (finasteride 5mg) vs. placebo.
- Aim was to examine the long-term benefit of finasteride symptomatic BPH.
- Key findings included:
- Prostate volume in placebo (+ 14%) and finasteride (-18%)
- Prostate volume in finasteride group reached nadir at 1 year and remained at this level
- Symptom score and flow rate in finasteride group showed modest and progressive improvements, in contrast to placebo group, which were unchanged
- Finasteride exhibited 57% reduction in risk of AUR and 55% of progression to surgery
- NNT for finasteride to prevent AUR = 25.

COMBINATION THERAPY

Combination therapy to treat LUTS associated with BPE refers to 5ARI + α-1 blocker.

NICE recommends combination therapy for men with:

- Moderate-to-severe LUTS, and
- Prostates estimated > 30g in size or PSA > 1.4ng/mL.

VIVA | The BPH station of the FRCS (Urol) viva is renowned to be the one where the most papers/studies need to be learned and quoted by distinction-level candidates. I recommend you familiarise yourself with all the papers I have included in this section by also reading the full publication online.

KEY PAPER | MTOPS (2003) [19]

- MTOPS stands for Medical Therapy of Prostatic Symptoms.
- Double-blind placebo-controlled study assessing impact of medical therapy on BPH progression (> 4-point rise in IPSS, development of AUR) mean follow-up 4.5 years.
- 3,000+ men (mean prostate volume 36mL) randomised to (placebo) vs. (doxazosin 8mg/day) vs. (finasteride 5mg/day) vs. (combination doxazosin + finasteride).
- Found that combination therapy provided benefits over either drug as monotherapy in terms of reduction in the risk of clinical progression.

KEY PAPER | CombAT (2008) [20]

- CombAT (COMBination of Avodart and Tamsulosin) where Avodart is dutasteride.
- 4-year, multi-centre, randomised, double-blind study.
- 4,800+ men aged ≥ 50 years with clinical diagnosis of BPH, IPSS > 12, randomised to (tamsulosin 400µg/day) vs. (dutasteride 0.5mg/day) vs. (combination of both).
- Key findings included:
- Combination superior to tamsulosin monotherapy but not dutasteride monotherapy at reducing the relative risk of AUR or BPH-related surgery
- Combination superior to both monotherapies at reducing RR of BPH progression
- Combination provided greater symptom benefit than either monotherapy at 4 years.

KEY PAPER | CONDUCT (2015) [21]

- 2-year multi-centre, randomised trial published in *BJUI*.
- 700+ men, with treatment-naive BPH, IPSS (8–19), prostate > 30g, PSA > 1.5ng/mL.
- Randomised to (combination 0.5mg dutasteride + 0.4mg tamsulosin) vs. WW.
- Key findings included:
    - Change in IPSS significantly greater for combination arm compared to WW
    - Risk of BPH progression reduced in combination group by 43%.

PHYTOTHERAPY

Phytotherapy (plant extracts) represent an alternative treatment for BPE.

The extracts of the same plant produced by different companies do not necessarily have the same biological or clinical effects, limiting ability to extrapolate benefit seen in one brand to others.

Options include: saw palmetto, Urtica dioica (stinging nettle), Pygeum Africanum.

NICE does not recommend offering phytotherapy to treat LUTS in men. [22]

SURGICAL TREATMENT

Surgical options to treat LUTS due to BPE should be considered in the following circumstances:

- Symptoms refractory to medical therapy (or medication not tolerated)
- HPCRU
- Recurrent AUR
- Elevated PVR or concomitant bladder stones
- Recurrent VH of proven prostatic origin, refractory to 5ARI therapy.

A key aspect to determine is whether patient wishes to preserve natural fertility.

The patient ideally should be counselled about all options such that he can make an informed choice.

TURP

TURP involves removing tissue from the transition zone of the prostate (TUIP involves incising the bladder outlet without tissue removal).

Bipolar TURP has similar efficacy but lower peri-operative morbidity compared to monopolar TURP.

EAU 2024 recommends offering mono- or bipolar TURP for the following: [23]

- Moderate-to-severe LUTS in men with prostate size 30–80mL.

Efficacy

TURP confers 90% chance of symptom improvement in BPE causing BOO – voiding symptoms improve faster than storage symptoms.

Improvements include Qmax (+162%), IPSS (-70%) and PVR (-77%).

Side-effects

The risks of TURP surgery include:

- Early: blood transfusion (1%), sepsis (≤ 3%) anaesthesia related, DVT/PE, TUR syndrome
- Late: urinary incontinence (rare), retrograde ejaculation (≤ 100%), ED (10%), stricture and re-do surgery (cumulative risk 2%/year, i.e. 10% at 5 years).

HoLEP

The holmium: yttrium-aluminium-garnet (Ho:YAG) LASER can be used to treat BOO.

Functions as solid-state LASER absorbed by prostate tissue, with the created heat (> 100°C) causing tissue vaporisation whilst coagulating blood vessels.

The irrigation fluid used for HoLEP is normal saline.

When directly compared to TURP, HoLEP demonstrates:

- Similar mid- to long-term efficacy
- Similar short-term safety and comparable rates of ED and retrograde ejaculation
- Longer operative times, shorter catheterisation and hospitalisation times.

HoLEP is supported by NICE and EAU 2024 – no cut-off prostate size is quoted; however, prostates are generally recommended to be > 80g in size.

UROLIFT®

Encroaching lateral lobes are compressed by small permanent implants under cystoscopic guidance, thus resulting in an opening of the prostatic urethra.

Do not perform UroLift® on patients with large obstructing median lobe (i.e. perform diagnostic flexible cystoscopy prior to offering this option).

Procedure can be done under local or general anaesthesia.

UroLift® has a low incidence of sexual side-effects and preserves ejaculatory function.

It improves LUTS and QOL, but not as much as TURP or HoLEP.

NICE 2021 recommends that UroLift® can be used for the treatment of male LUTS: [24]

- As alternative to TURP and HoLEP
- Patients aged ≥ 50 years
- Prostate volume 30–80mL.

EAU 2024 recommends offering UroLift® to treat LUTS:

- In men interested in preserving ejaculatory function
- Prostate volume < 70mL
- No middle lobe.

| **KEY PAPER** | L.I.F.T. Study (2017) [25] |

- Multi-centre, randomised controlled trial for LUTS patients with 5-year follow-up.
- Included men aged > 50 years, with IPSS > 12, $Q_{max} \leq 12$mL/s, prostate volume 30–80mL.
- Randomised 2:1 to (UroLift®) vs. (blinded sham control).
- Outcome assessment IPSS, Q_{max}, QOL, adverse events.
- Key findings included:
- IPSS improvement was 88% greater than sham at 3 months
- Benefits durable at 5 years with improvements in IPSS (36%), QOL (50%) and Q_{max} (44%).

REZUM®

The REZUM® system uses thermal energy in the form of water vapour to induce cell necrosis.

Performed as day case; however, patients should be discharged home with catheter in situ.

Currently there is no RCT comparing REZUM® with UroLift®, which is its likely competitor.

NICE 2020 recommends that REZUM® can be used to treat LUTS caused by BPE: [26]

- Moderate-to-severe LUTS (IPSS $\geq$ 13)
- Prostate volume 30–80mL.

EAU 2024 does not make a recommendation on its use.

PROSTATE ARTERY EMBOLISATION

PAE can be performed as day case under local anaesthesia, with access via femoral/radial arteries.

Tiny plastic beads are injected to lead to cell infarction/death and volume reduction.

Patient should have CT angiogram before the procedure – severe atherosclerosis may rule out PAE as an option, although it can be performed unilaterally with likely lower success rates.

Risks of PAE include:

- Infection, bruising or bleeding at the puncture site or in urine
- Allergy to contrast
- Abandoning procedure if vessels are found to be too small or diseased to treat
- Post-embolisation syndrome (e.g. flu-like symptoms, nausea)
- Ischaemic damage to bladder, bowel, penis.

NICE 2018 supports PAE to treat BPH provided: [27]

- Performed by interventional radiologist with specific training and expertise in the procedure
- Patient selection should be done by a urologist and interventional radiologist.

EAU 2024 recommends PAE to treat moderate-to-severe LUTS provided:

- Patient accepts less optimal outcomes compared to TURP
- It is being performed in a unit where urologists and interventional radiologists collaborate in patient selection and follow-up.

KEY PAPER ROPE Study (2018) [28]

- Multi-centre UK study to assess PAE safety + efficacy in treating LUTS and compare to TURP.
- 305 patients included: PAE (n=216) and TURP (n=89), followed up to 12 months.
- Primary outcomes were improvements in IPSS and complication data.
- Key findings included:
- PAE was clinically effective (median improvement of 10 points on IPSS at 12 months)
- PAE not as effective as TURP
- PAE was safe and associated with faster return to normal activities compared to TURP.

AQUABLATION®

Aquablation® uses hydro-dissection to ablate prostatic parenchyma while sparing collagenous structures such as blood vessels and capsule.

Targeted high-velocity saline ablates prostatic tissue without generating thermal energy (heat-free).

Procedure is done with combined endoscopic and TRUS view, procedure is done in automated manner robotically and the treatment duration is independent of prostate size.

The ablated tissue is aspirated through ports in the handpiece.

The technology is approved by NICE.

EAU 2024 recommends offering Aquablation® to treat moderate-to-severe LUTS:

- Prostate volume 30–80mL
- Provided patients are informed that there is a lack of long-term follow-up data.

VIVA Many candidates may not have performed or seen Aquablation® before, and indeed currently may not have the opportunity to see it live in the operating theatre. I recommend you watch online videos to familiarise yourself with how the procedure is done.

> **KEY PAPER** | WATER Trial (2018) [29]
>
> - Double-blind, multi-centre RCT for patients with moderate-to-severe LUTS due to BPH.
> - 181 patients randomised to (TURP) vs. (Aquablation®), with aim of comparing efficacy (via IPSS) and safety outcomes (via Clavien–Dindo) at 6 months.
> - Key findings included:
> - Aquablation® was non-inferior to TURP in IPSS benefit at 6 months
> - Aquablation® had a lower associated risk of sexual dysfunction.

iTIND®

The iTIND® is a nitinol basket which under direct visualisation is deployed inside the prostate in expanded configuration, to compress obstructing tissue.

The basket exerts radial force causing ischaemic necrosis.

Patient is discharged as day case and brought back for basket removal after 5–7 days.

Long-term data is limited; EAU 2024 does not offer recommendation for its use.

Currently the PREMISE trial is ongoing:

- PREMISE (Prostate Resection versus Minimally Invasive Surgery Evaluation)
- RCT comparing iTIND® vs. REZUM® vs. UroLift® vs. TURP.

HIGH-PRESSURE CHRONIC RETENTION OF URINE

HPCRU is an indication for urgent urethral catheterisation and subsequent BOO surgery.

Post-obstructive diuresis requires close monitoring of potassium, with an IV saline replacement of 2/3 of the volume of the previous hourly urine output.

Post-obstructive diuresis occurs physiologically due to fluid/electrolyte accumulation.

Diuresis is defined as > 200mL/hour of urine output for 2 hours or more.

Pathological elements of diuresis include:

- Poor response of collecting ducts to ADH

- Increased production of ANP

- Inability to maintain medullary solute gradient due to increased blood flow

- Defective medullary solute gradient (reduced NaCl and urea reabsorption).

HPCRU ensues gradually over time, as the bladder retains an ever-greater amount of urine after voiding, resulting in an *end void pressure*.

The patient's bladder fills and the pressure rises until they void (end fill pressure) after which the pressure drops down to end void pressure again.

Only relief of the obstruction will bring the resting bladder pressure down (Image 6).

Image 6 – Graphical demonstration of bladder pressures in HPCRU

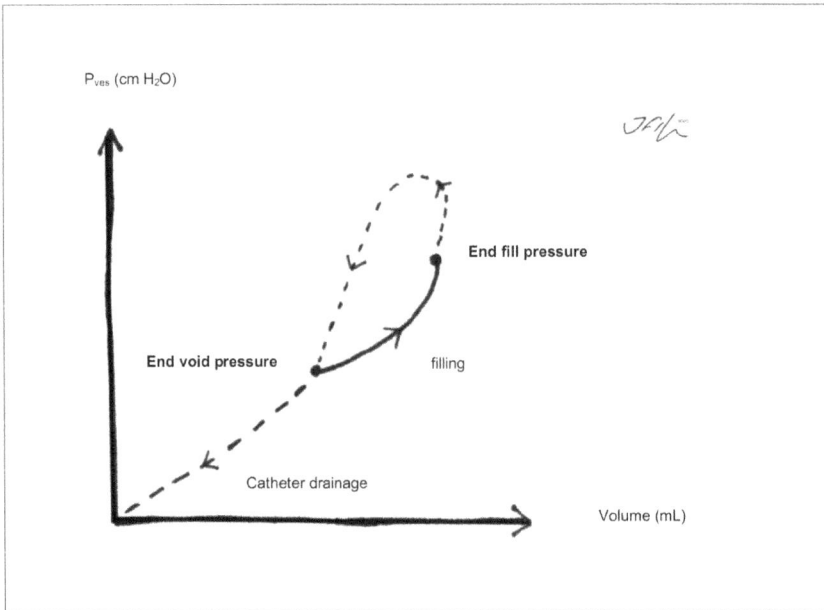

GFR takes ≤ 3 months to fully recover (plasma creatinine continues to decrease during period).

Recall that creatinine is excreted by tubules as well as through glomerular filtration, therefore tubular function recovers within 14 days but full glomerular function can take 3 months.

About 80% of creatinine clearance is due to GFR and 20% to renal tubular secretion.

Thus creatinine clearance is an over-estimate of actual GFR (i.e. becomes important in renal failure where tubular secretion may be responsible for relatively greater proportion of clearance).

99mTc DTPA (diethylene-triamine-penta-acetic acid) clearance is another means of calculating GFR.

VARICOCELE

A varicocele is an abnormal dilatation of the veins in the pampiniform plexus of the spermatic cord, which is formed from internal spermatic and gonadal veins.

EPIDEMIOLOGY

Varicoceles present in ≤ 25% of male population, and 25% of men with abnormal semen parameters.

Rare prior to puberty, and the incidence rises with increasing age.

AETIOLOGY

90% of varicoceles feature on the left side, which therefore proposes reasons for its development:

- Left testicular vein drains into left renal vein, higher pressure system
- Absence of venous valves is more commonly found on the left side
- Left renal vein may be compressed between superior mesenteric artery and aorta.

There appears to be a correlation between varicocele and infertility.

One theory relates to counter-current mechanism for heat exchange provided by pampiniform plexus to arteries entering testes, which is impaired by the varicocele.

This may result in increased scrotal temperature and reflux of toxic metabolites.

CLASSIFICATION

Varicoceles are graded according to findings on physical examination (Table 16).

Table 16 – Grading of varicoceles

Grade	Description
0	Sub-clinical (seen on US only)
1	Palpable on Valsalva manoeuvre only
2	Palpable on standing, not visible
3	Palpable and visible

DIAGNOSTIC EVALUATION

The factors present in the patient history may include:

- Heavy, dragging sensation in scrotum
- Symptoms affected with position.

Patient examination with consent and in the presence of a chaperone should assess for:

- Palpable *bag of worms* in the scrotum
- Repeat examination in lying and standing position
- Assess ipsilateral testicular volume (often reduced)
- Palpate ipsilateral kidney.

The imaging of choice is *scrotal Doppler US* (ensure to scan ipsilateral kidney).

MANAGEMENT

Most patients with varicoceles do not need or wish to undergo any treatment.

NICE 2023 [30] recommends urology referral to consider surgery in the following:

- Grade 2 or 3 varicocele which is symptomatic
- Grade 2 or 3 varicocele with abnormal semen parameters in man wishing to be fertile
- Grade 2 or 3 varicocele in an adolescent with ipsilateral testicular growth arrest.

IR embolisation (coils or sclerosing agents) has high success rates; patients must be counselled regarding recurrence after embolisation, shrinkage of testicle and risk of sub-fertility.

Surgically the spermatic/testicular vein can be clipped laparoscopically or via microsurgical techniques (likely preferable option for patients being treated in context of infertility).

Open surgical options include via inguinal (Ivanissevich) or high-retro-peritoneal (Palomo) approaches.

Improvement in semen parameters are seen in 70% of men undergoing surgical intervention.

KEY PAPER | Evers and Collins (2004) [31]

- Meta-analysis evaluating effect of varicocele treatment on pregnancy rates in sub-fertile couples.

- Concluded that varicocele treatment did not improve pregnancy rates.

- Limitations were the inclusion of patients with sub-clinical varicoceles and normal semen parameters (when these were excluded, 36% (treated) vs. 20% (untreated)).

REFERENCES

1. McNeal JE (1981). The zonal anatomy of the prostate. *Prostate*, *2*(1), 35–49.
2. Bartsch G, Rittmaster RS, Klocker H (2000). Dihydrotestosterone and the concept of 5alpha-reductase inhibition in human benign prostatic hyperplasia. *European Urology*, *37*(4), 367–380.
3. Rittmaster R, Hahn RG, Ray P, et al. (2008). Effect of dutasteride on intraprostatic androgen levels in men with benign prostatic hyperplasia or prostate cancer. *Urology*, *72*(4), 808–812.
4. Althof SE, McMahon CG, Waldinger MD, et al. (2014). An update of the International Society of Sexual Medicine's guidelines for the diagnosis and treatment of premature ejaculation (PE). *Journal of Sexual Medicine*, *11*(6), 1,392–1,422.
5. https://www.baus.org.uk/_userfiles/pages/files/Patients/Leaflets/Vasectomy.pdf [accessed 18 May 2020].
6. Grey BR, Thompson A, Jenkins BL, et al. (2012). UK practice regarding reversal of vasectomy 2001–2010: relevance to best contemporary patient management. *BJU International*, *110*(7), 1,040–1,047.
7. Van Dongen J, Tekle FB, van Roijen H (2012). Pregnancy rate after vasectomy reversal in a contemporary series: influence of smoking, semen quality and post-surgical use of assisted reproductive techniques. *BJUI International*, *110*(4), 562–567.
8. Kalsi JS, Minhas S, Muneer A (2018). Andrology. In: Arya M, Shergill I, Fernando HS, et al., *Viva Practice for the FRCS (Urol) and Postgraduate Urology Examinations*, second edition, CRC Press, London.
9. https://commons.wikimedia.org/wiki/File:Penis_cross_section.svg [last accessed 18 August 2024].
10. Rosen RC, Cappelleri JC, Smith MD, et al. (1999). Development and evaluation of an abridged, 5-item version of the International Index of Erectile Function (IIEF-5) as a diagnostic tool for erectile dysfunction. *International Journal of Impotence Research*, *11*(6), 319–326.
11. Salonia A, Bettocchi C, Capogrosso P, et al. (2024). EAU Guidelines on Sexual and Reproductive Health. Available at: https://d56bochluxqnz.cloudfront.net/documents/full-guideline/EAU-Guidelines-on-Sexual-and-Reproductive-Health-2024_2024-05-23-101205_nmbi.pdf [last accessed 10 September 2024].
12. Hackett G, Kirby M, Edwards D, et al. (2017). British Society for Sexual Medicine guidelines on adult testosterone deficiency, with statements for UK practice. *Journal of Sexual Medicine*, *14*(12), 1,504–1,523.

13. Cooper TG, Noonan E, Von Eckardstein S, et al. (2010). World Health Organization reference values for human semen characteristics. *Human Reproduction Update, 16*(3), 231–245.

14. Chung E, Atmoko W, Saleh R, et al. (2024). Sixth edition of the World Health Organization laboratory manual of semen analysis: Updates and essential take away for busy clinicians. *Arab Journal of Urology, 22*(2), 71–74.

15. Weidner W, Hauck EW, Schnitker J, et al. (2005). Potassium paraaminobenzoate (POTABA™) in the treatment of Peyronie's disease: a prospective, placebo-controlled, randomized study. *European Urology, 47*(4), 530–536.

16. Barrett-Harlow B, Wang R (2016). Oral therapy for Peyronie's disease, does it work? *Translational Andrology and Urology, 5*(3), 296.

17. Jacobsen SJ, Jacobson DJ, Girman CJ, et al. (1999). Treatment for benign prostatic hyperplasia among community dwelling men: the Olmsted County study of urinary symptoms and health status. *Journal of Urology, 162*(4), 1,301–1,306.

18. Roehrborn CG, Bruskewitz R, Nickel GC, et al. (2000). Urinary retention in patients with BPH treated with finasteride or placebo over 4 years. *European Urology, 37*(5), 528–536.

19. McConnell JD, Roehrborn CG, Bautista OM, et al. (2003). The long-term effect of doxazosin, finasteride, and combination therapy on the clinical progression of benign prostatic hyperplasia. *New England Journal of Medicine, 349*(25), 2,387–2,398.

20. Roehrborn CG, Siami P, Barkin J (2008). The effects of dutasteride, tamsulosin and combination therapy on lower urinary tract symptoms in men with benign prostatic hyperplasia and prostatic enlargement: 2-year results from the CombAT study. *Journal of Urology, 179*(2), 616–621.

21. Roehrborn CG, Oyarzabal Perez I, Roos EP (2015). Efficacy and safety of a fixed-dose combination of dutasteride and tamsulosin treatment (Duodart®) compared with watchful waiting with initiation of tamsulosin therapy if symptoms do not improve, both provided with lifestyle advice, in the management of treatment-naïve men with moderately symptomatic benign prostatic hyperplasia: 2-year CONDUCT study results. *BJU International, 116*(3), 450–459.

22. NICE Guidelines – Lower urinary tract symptoms in men: management. Available at: https://www.nice.org.uk/guidance/cg97/resources/lower-urinary-tract-symptoms-in-men-management-pdf-975754394053 [last accessed 15 September 2024].

23. Corbu JN, Gacci M, Hashim H, et al. (2024). EAU Guidelines on Management of Non-Neurogenic Male Lower Urinary Tract Symptoms (LUTS). Available at: https://d56bochluxqnz.cloudfront.net/documents/full-guideline/EAU-Guidelines-on-Non-Neurogenic-Male-LUTS-2024.pdf [last accessed 19 September 2024].

24. NICE Guidelines – UroLift for treating lower urinary tract symptoms of benign prostatic hyperplasia. Available at: https://www.nice.org.uk/guidance/mtg58/resources/urolift-for-treating-lower-urinary-tract-symptoms-of-benign-prostatic-hyperplasia-pdf-64372122962629 [last accessed 20 September 2024].

25. Roehrborn CG, Barkin J, Gange SN, et al. (2017). Five year results of the prospective randomised controlled prostatic urethral L.I.F.T. study. *Canadian Journal of Urology*, *24*(3), 8,802–8,813.

26. NICE Guidelines – Rezum for treating lower urinary tract symptoms secondary to benign prostatic hyperplasia. Available at: https://www.nice.org.uk/guidance/mtg49/resources/rezum-for-treating-lower-urinary-tract-symptoms-secondary-to-benign-prostatic-hyperplasia-pdf-64372064176069 [last accessed 20 September 2024].

27. NICE Guidelines – Prostate artery embolisation for lower urinary tract symptoms caused by benign prostatic hyperplasia. Available at: https://www.nice.org.uk/guidance/ipg611/resources/prostate-artery-embolisation-for-lower-urinary-tract-symptoms-caused-by-benign-prostatic-hyperplasia-pdf-1899873917137861 [last accessed 20 September 2024].

28. Ray AF, Powell J, Speakman MJ, et al. (2018). Efficacy and safety of prostate artery embolisation for benign prostatic hyperplasia: an observational study and propensity-matched comparison with transurethral resection of the prostate (the UK-ROPE study). *BJU International*, *122*(2), 270–282.

29. Gilling P, Barber N, Bidair M, et al. (2018). WATER: A Double-Blind, Randomised, Controlled Trial of Aquablation® vs Transurethral Resection of the Prostate in Benign Prostatic Hyperplasia. *Journal of Urology*, *199*(5), 1,252–1,261.

30. NICE. Scenario: Management of varicocele. Available at: https://cks.nice.org.uk/topics/varicocele/management/management/ [last accessed 20 September 2024].

31. Evers JL, Collins J (2004). Surgery or embolisation for varicocele in subfertile men. *Cochrane Database of Systematic Reviews*, (3).

ANDROLOGY & BPH MCQS

1. Which of the following is the only SSRI licensed for on-demand use to treat premature ejaculation?

   A) Paroxetine
   B) Fluoxetine
   C) Sertraline
   D) Dapoxetine
   E) Fluvoxamine

2. What is the BAUS quoted figure for early failure rate after vasectomy?

   A) 1/200
   B) 1/250
   C) 1/300
   D) 1/350
   E) 1/400

3. What is the BAUS quoted figure for late failure rate after vasectomy?

   A) 1/2,000
   B) 1/2,500
   C) 1/3,000
   D) 1/3,500
   E) None of the above

4. Which of the following arteries does not normally supply the prostate gland?

   A) Inferior vesical artery
   B) Posterior division of internal iliac artery
   C) Middle rectal artery
   D) Internal pudendal artery
   E) All of the above supply the prostate

5. Which of the following semen analysis results would allow the patient to be given special clearance following vasectomy?

   A) $< 10^3$ immotile sperm, 14 weeks after vasectomy
   B) $< 10^4$ immotile sperm, 14 weeks after vasectomy
   C) $< 10^5$ immotile sperm, 14 weeks after vasectomy
   D) $< 10^6$ immotile sperm, 14 weeks after vasectomy
   E) None of the above

6. Which of the following questions does not feature in the SHIM questionnaire to evaluate ED?

   A) How do you rate your confidence that you could keep an erection?
   B) When you had erections with sexual stimulation, how often were your erections hard enough for penetration?
   C) How often were you able to initiate an erection at the start of sexual activity?
   D) When you attempted sex, how often was it satisfactory for you?
   E) During sex, how difficult was it to maintain your erection to completion of intercourse?

7. Which of the following is considered a likely normal peak systolic velocity on penile colour Doppler for assessing ED?

   A) > 5cm/s
   B) > 10cm/s
   C) > 20cm/s
   D) > 25cm/s
   E) None of the above

8. What are the standard recommended daily doses of vardenafil in mg?

   A) 10, 20, 30
   B) 25, 50, 100
   C) 10, 20, 40
   D) 5, 10, 20
   E) 2, 5, 10

9. Which of the following would be a standard dose (in µg) of on-demand MUSE® inserted as pellet into the urethra?

   A) 50
   B) 100
   C) 200
   D) 250
   E) 500

10. What is the half-life of sildenafil (in hours)?

   A) 2
   B) 4
   C) 6
   D) 8
   E) 10

11. *Approximately 50% of testosterone is metabolised via the conjugation process into which of the following breakdown products?*

    A) Testosterone glucuronide
    B) Dihydrotestosterone
    C) Testosterone nitrate
    D) Androsterone
    E) 3α-etiocholanediol

12. *Which of the following is formed at completion of second meiotic division in spermatogenesis?*

    A) Secondary spermatocyte
    B) Spermatid
    C) Primary spermatocyte
    D) Spermatozoa
    E) None of the above

13. *Which of the following is the lower limit of normal value for total sperm count, on a man's semen analysis investigation, as per WHO (fifth and sixth editions) criteria?*

    A) 27×10^6
    B) 33×10^6
    C) 39×10^6
    D) 45×10^6
    E) 51×10^6

14. *Which of the following is the lower limit of normal value for sperm morphology (% normal forms), on a man's semen analysis investigation, as per WHO (fifth and sixth editions) criteria?*

    A) 1%
    B) 3%
    C) 5%
    D) 7%
    E) None of the above

15. *Which of the following is activated in the inflammatory response following tissue injury, which is a contributing factor to development of fibrosis resulting in Peyronie's disease?*

    A) TGF-β
    B) TGF-α
    C) TGF-δ
    D) IFN-α
    E) IFN-β

16. *Which of the following is supported by EAU 2024 as an intra-lesional treatment option for Peyronie's disease?*

    A) Betamethasone
    B) Botulinum toxin
    C) IFN-β
    D) POTABA
    E) None of the above

17. *If a man is being evaluated for non-neurogenic LUTS, what is the probability of underlying obstruction if the patient's Q_{max} on uroflowmetry is 13mL/s?*

    A) 40%
    B) 50%
    C) 60%
    D) 70%
    E) 80%

18. *What is the correct lower limit of normal for Q_{max} on uroflowmetry for a healthy female patient aged 60 years?*

    A) > 12mL/s
    B) > 14mL/s
    C) > 16mL/s
    D) > 18mL/s
    E) > 20mL/s

19. *What does T100 refer to on a uroflowmetry test?*

    A) Time to void first 100mL of urine
    B) Total voiding time including interruptions
    C) Presence of prolonged voiding time beyond 100 seconds
    D) Voiding time following Q_{max}
    E) T100 is not applicable to a standard uroflowmetry test

20. *What is the correct lower limit of normal for Q_{max} on uroflowmetry for a healthy male patient aged 65 years?*

    A) > 11mL/s
    B) > 13mL/s
    C) > 15mL/s
    D) > 17mL/s
    E) > 19mL/s

21. *Above which PSA value is considered an independent risk factor for progressing to acute urinary retention in a male patient with LUTS?*

    A) PSA > 1.0ng/mL
    B) PSA > 1.2ng/mL
    C) PSA > 1.4ng/mL
    D) PSA > 1.6ng/mL
    E) PSA > 1.8ng/mL

22. *In the Olmsted County Study, what was found to be the mean yearly increase in IPSS points?*

    A) 0.18 points/year
    B) 0.22 points/year
    C) 0.26 points/year
    D) 0.30 points/year
    E) 0.34 points/year

23. *What were the treatment arms in the CombAT trial?*

    A) Tamsulosin vs. WW
    B) Dutasteride vs. WW
    C) Tamsulosin vs. dutasteride
    D) Tamsulosin vs. dutasteride vs. placebo
    E) None of the above

24. *Which of the following symptoms does not feature on the IPSS questionnaire?*

    A) Urgency
    B) Intermittency
    C) Nocturia
    D) Hesitancy
    E) Incomplete emptying

25. *Which of the following is not a risk factor for developing acute urinary retention in a male patient with LUTS?*

    A) IPSS > 5
    B) $Q_{max} < 12mL/s$
    C) Prostate volume > 30mL
    D) Age > 70 years
    E) None of the above

BONUS CHAPTER
VIVA TIPS
& TRICKS

GENERAL ADVICE

Once you have cleared Section 1 (the written part) of the FRCS (Urol) examination, you will hopefully be reassured to hear that you have completed the harder leg of the journey! The written exam always has an element of the unknown to it and it is difficult to know with confidence when you are truly "ready" to sit it. Revising for Section 1 is also more of a solitary experience, with many late candle-lit nights spent pouring over books and guidelines trying to memorise TNM staging and percentages.

Section 2 (the viva), however, is a totally different (and arguably better) experience. All the factual knowledge that you already have which carried you through Section 1 must now sublimate into spoken words – other skills such as good body language, clear, logical and concise thinking and diction, the ability to prioritise and critically appraise information all come into play. Knowledge alone unfortunately will not carry you through the Section 2 viva and in truth good communication and presentation skills are almost equally important.

Inevitably some candidates are naturally stronger than others in these domains, but what holds true for everyone is that practise, practise, practise is key. If you try to venture alone simply with your textbooks, you will most likely fail. On the other hand, if you form a productive and positive small revision group and practise (almost) every day for the 6–8 weeks leading up to your exam, as well as attend the relevant revision courses, you will very likely pass.

Revision Group

I recommend that your revision group should ideally have three or four people – more than this may well lead to a situation of "too many urologists spoil the broth" – some will become more vocal contributors and others more silent, which does not help either party.

Two people are insufficient as you will always be playing off each other and never able to observe as a third party, which in itself is an important part of practising.

A group of four is helpful as it allows you to split into groups of two when you meet as a team, and between four urologists you are likely to have a spread of different sub-speciality interests amongst yourselves, as we all naturally have stronger areas which we can help other members with and weaker areas where we can benefit by learning from them.

My team had an agreement that every evening around 9pm we would by default practise on a group video-conference call. Inevitably, with hospital on-calls and family commitments, the odd person may miss out occasionally, but our formal agreement helped with consistency and discipline. Online sessions were effective to a degree, but closer to the exam we met regularly in coffee shops or in each other's houses, as you need to be face-to-face to simulate true viva body language and time pressure. Make sure you time each viva you practise and the observers should provide helpful feedback.

Along with all your group, try to each organise a viva session with a consultant sub-specialist in your respective hospitals and invite the others to join. That way you will experience different viva techniques including from senior colleagues that you may never have met before, which simulates the exam where, by and large, you will be tested by senior colleagues you do not know.

Revision Timings

I do not recommend intense viva practice before the BAUS FRCS (Urol) revision course – your revision sessions will likely be unstructured and inefficient. Attending the course will give you clarity on the viva structure and technique – such that your subsequent viva practice sessions will be much more effective and worthwhile thereafter.

Provided you practise regularly, there is plenty of time after the course to make yourself exam-ready.

Rather, in the two weeks leading up to the BAUS FRCS (Urol) course, I would recommend that you go through the entire syllabus again with your textbooks, so that your knowledge is refreshed and you will make the most of the lectures, which will then serve as fine-tuning of your knowledge and revision notes.

Viva "Flow"

The viva is not a friendly chat with a cup of tea in a drawing room, as perhaps once upon a time it was made out to be.

The examiners have a job to do, which is to put you at ease and try to get you through the full scenario so you can maximise your marks. They will not mislead you and if you make a mistake, they are instructed to not lead candidates up the garden path and dig you into a deeper hole. They are also advised to be as deadpan as possible, so do not expect particular encouragement or commendation when you are doing well or frowns and eye-rolling if you are doing badly.

The "flow" of the viva is a term (fitting with urology itself) that you will often hear across revision courses and practice sessions with FRCS (Urol) positive colleagues. The scenario is a story which has a beginning, middle and end – your aim being to progress through at a steady pace such that you complete it in good time.

Getting the flow right is not easy, but it will come with practice.

Some questions – perhaps even the opening one to the station – might actually be closed type questions, for example: *"What is the absolute 5-year survival benefit of neo-adjuvant chemotherapy prior to radical cystectomy?"* Answer this concisely: *"5% improvement"* or better still *"the ABC trial found a 5% benefit in 5-year survival"*.

And leave it at that. It is clearly a closed question and so do not make unnecessary extra conversation that will cost you time and not gain you marks. By clearly closing your answer, you allow the examiner to move on and maintain the flow.

Other questions are clearly open and require broader answers, for example: *"How would you assess this patient with LUTS?"* or *"Discuss the evidence favouring the active treatment of staghorn calculi".*

Here, having a structured approach to your answers will serve you well – and I will detail a few helpful strategies later. As a rule of thumb, if you notice yourself talking continuously for several minutes then something probably isn't right (the examiners may not interrupt you); and likewise, an abrupt early finish on your behalf may feel on the examiner's side of the table like the handbrake of a car in motion has just been pulled, which is certainly converse to having smooth flow.

If you forget or do not know the answer, think for a few seconds before the silence gets too deafening, and then state "I am sorry, I do not recall this" – and move on. Keep the flow. You are also likely to remain more positive, as a long, interminable pause with still no answer at the end of it will knock your confidence. Paradoxically, being "confident" in not being able to answer a particular question may come across as being aware of your limitations, which is certainly preferable to appearing uncertain, lacking confidence and hesitant.

As it happens, you may in fact come back to the answer later if it does slip into your mind and claim the marks anyway.

Neuro-linguistic Programming

Neuro-linguistic programming is an approach to communication that looks at how our (and with relevance to you, how your examiner's) brains interpret the signals he/she receives.

Gold-medal winners no doubt have sound knowledge (I have practised with five to date), but more likely they are regularly hitting full marks because of the way they are coming across to the examiners, aided by their body language, communication skills, confidence and personable demeanour.

A golden mantra for the viva is: "If you walk in as a consultant, you will walk out as a consultant" – and that definitely holds true. The bar to pass the exam is to answer at a level expected from a day-one DGH consultant urologist, and so you should act like one. This is easier said than done, as you probably have spent many years as a resident doctor and none as a consultant, but try to slowly get in the mindset through your practice sessions.

Walk into the examination room with your head held high, sit down, smile to the examiners, lean forward slightly (thus appearing interested) and maintain eye contact with <u>both</u> examiners (only one will talk to you, the other will be marking). Have a strategy of keeping your hands under control, as nerves can make you over-gesticulate, doodle with your pen or scratch your nose, all of which can be distracting. As my baseline safety position, I personally hold my hands together by interlocking my fingers and rest them on the edge of the table, so they are in view and protecting each other from wandering away.

Small, subtle but persistent clues in your communication to your examiners will convey a sense of consultant authority as opposed to junior-doctor deference. Be careful, of course, to be suitably confident but not arrogant. The following list is not exhaustive but should get your mind thinking:

- Rather than saying *"I could do this"* or *"In my trust we do that"*, refer to *"in <u>my</u> practice"* e.g. *"in my practice I perform a retrograde before stenting a ureter"*.

- Garner help from other consultant colleagues in complex or unwell patient scenarios, and refer to them as your own, which emulates being a practising consultant in a hospital known and liked by his/her colleagues e.g. *"I will first liaise with my trusted consultant colleague anaesthetist regarding this patient's mortality risk from surgery, and then call my microbiology consultant colleague to confirm the optimal choice of antibiotics"*.

- Refer to clinics/theatres as *"my one-stop LUTS clinic"* or *"I would undertake this radical inguinal orchidectomy on my next elective operating list"* – which suggests you do and are in control of your own work, rather than delegating to others.

- Rather than delegating a decision to an MDT, show confident but safe decision-making initiative by suggesting what you would do but accepting that other colleagues' views also matter, and therefore rephrase to: *"I believe this 50-year-old man with intermediate risk localised prostate cancer would benefit from radical prostatectomy. I would therefore personally list him* (pro-active behaviour hint) *for discussion in my local uro-oncology MDT, proposing* (pro-active word) *this option and seeking opinion from my colleagues, recognising that alternative options such as radical radiotherapy or active surveillance may be considered"*.

- In a given patient scenario, clearly voice your relevant concerns/clinical priorities early on, as a consultant recognises the nuances of given clinical scenarios and prioritises these: e.g. *"I am worried that this patient is septic, therefore I will do…"* or *"I know that lymph-node involvement is the most important prognostic factor in penile cancer, and so I will…"*.

- Be aware of your day-one DGH consultant limitations. Whilst of course for TURP, URS, and circumcision, for example, you should complete these yourself independently, you are not expected to do a neobladder on your first day as a consultant on your own, so it would be perfectly acceptable to say: *"I would undertake a neobladder on my operating list, and organise for my senior colleague pelvic oncologist to be present for dual consultant operating and support"*.

I strongly recommend that you listen to colleagues who score well in the BAUS FRCS (Urol) revision course and reflect on what tools or soundbites they are consistently using that clearly the examiners like to hear.

In your revision groups I would also focus on critiquing each other to develop more confident and authoritative-sounding communication.

Other favourable sub-conscious clues you can regularly give your examiner, which will likely help you, include appearing to be:

- Pro-active (*"I will do the arterial blood gas without delay…"*)

- Polite and pleasant (*"I will introduce myself and welcome them into my LUTS clinic where I will take a focused urological history"*)

- Compassionate (*"I will tell the patient that I am very sorry they have testicular cancer, and explain they need to proceed to chemotherapy…"*)

- A team-player (*"I will manage this patient's metastatic cord compression by personally facilitating a multi-disciplinary approach working alongside oncology, neurosurgery and my Trust's metastatic cord-compression co-ordinator"*).

In essence, being nice, helpful, polite, compassionate and hard working is likely to get you far in life anyway – you just need to sub-consciously convey this to your examiner, whilst of course displaying your clinical and factual knowledge as well.

If you can also appear confident with all of this – you are onto a winner.

Final golden rule of the viva: do <u>not</u> ever argue with the examiner. You will always lose.

OPENING GAMBITS

Truth be told, within the first minute the examiners can likely tell whether this given candidate knows what he/she is doing or not, and once you have been silently labelled as good (or bad) in their minds, it is a harder task to shift opinions in either direction.

A good debut/opening gambit will really serve you well. You will come across as confident and well-practised, getting the viva flowing well and coherently.

Having a structure for opening gambits is important to protect you from nerves, as inevitably the most stressful moment of the station is the start of it, when you have first to say something, particularly as you do not know what is about to hit you – which is exactly the time when your opening gambit comes in to save you. From the examiners' perspective, their first impression of you is akin, sadly, to judging a book by its cover. We are all guilty of this as it is inherent human nature in an interview situation – but you need to get it right.

I recommend that you practise, practise, practise these opening gambits whenever they are appropriate to use. Indeed if you can create a better one of your own then use that by all means, but have consistency and a systematic approach in utilising it.

Out-patient Scenario

For any out-patient/non-emergent type of scenario, such as:

- You have been referred a 55-year-old man with a PSA of 10, how would you assess him?

  Or:

- The GP has referred you a 60-year-old man with a history of erectile dysfunction, tell me the key points in history and examination

I would recommend that you consider using the following structure:

1. Tell the examiner <u>where</u> you would see the patient and take ownership of that service (e.g. in my one-stop LUTS clinic or my dedicated ED clinic)

2. Tell the examiner on what <u>time basis</u> you would see the patient (e.g. routine, 2-week wait)

3. Tell the examiner <u>who else would be present</u> in the consulting room (e.g. uro-oncology nurse specialist, ED specialist nurse, or even patient's partner in infertility scenario, for example)

4. Tell the examiner what basic work-up/actions/tests you would do prior to them entering the consultation room (e.g. complete IPSS form, repeat PSA test, urine dipstick)

5. Then proceed to say *"I would then welcome the patient in and introduce myself* (i.e. marks for politeness) *and take a focused urological history…"* and take it from there.

The above examples of scenarios therefore become:

*   You have been referred a 55-year-old man with a PSA of 10, how would you assess him?

    "I would see this patient in my out-patient urology clinic (1) on a two-week wait basis (2), with my clinical nurse specialist present (3). Prior to him entering the consultation room (4) I would ensure he has repeated his PSA and had a urine dipstick. I would then welcome the patient in and introduce myself (5) and take a focused urological history…".

*   The GP has referred you a 60-year-old man with a history of erectile dysfunction, tell me the key points in history and examination.

    "I would see this patient in my dedicated ED clinic (1), on a routine basis (2), with my ED nurse specialist present (3). Prior to him entering the consultation room (4) I would ensure he has completed an IIEF-5 score and had an up-to-date early-morning testosterone, cholesterol and HBA1c. I would then welcome the patient in and introduce myself (5) and take a focused urological history…".

You can apply this five-step format to most out-patient scenarios you can think of and I believe it works effectively it getting the viva going at pace, with subtle clues to the examiner of your pro-activity, organisational skills and professional demeanour.

Emergency Scenario/Unwell Patient

To a certain degree you will have to mould your opening gambit in an emergency scenario, to reflect how unwell the patient is that you are presented with.

For example, a testicular torsion is clearly a very urgent scenario; however, it is extremely unlikely that the patient will be haemodynamically unstable as a result of the condition – so in this case an extensive "A-to-E assessment via CCrISP algorithm" is clearly not required.

Likewise, a polytrauma patient involved in a road-traffic accident who has a possible urethral injury will need more emphasis on the ATLS algorithm and ensuring their airway and c-spine are safe before the urologist worries about their urethra.

Take for example the following emergency scenarios:

- A+E calls you to see a 12-year-old boy with a short history of testicular pain

- The ward calls you about your patient, on whom you performed a TURP this afternoon, informing you that he is drowsy, febrile and his blood pressure is low.

As a rule of thumb, for any emergency scenario, I would suggest you follow this structure:

1. Tell the examiner that you <u>recognise the urgent nature</u> of the situation and better still, <u>state what is your main concern</u> of what might be going on (e.g. *"I recognise this is a potential urological emergency as this patient sounds like he might be suffering a post-operative bleed"*).

2. Tell the examiner you would see the patient yourself without delay.

3. Tell the examiner that on arrival you would introduce yourself and undertake a systematic A-to-E assessment following the CCrISP algorithm.

   - If the scenario does not involve a haemodynamically unstable patient, you can say (3) quickly and proceed with: *"providing his vital parameters were within normal range, I would proceed to take a focused urological history"*.

   - If the scenario does involve a haemodynamically unstable patient, then you may have to describe the A-to-E components in more detail, stating for example how much oxygen you would give, IVI resuscitation etc. and only proceeding to taking a focused urological history once the patient is more stable.

- If the patient is febrile and potentially septic as well, make sure you state that in addition to the above you would ensure that all facets of the Sepsis-6 bundle have been completed.
- Likewise a trauma patient may require you to detail the steps of the ATLS algorithm in more detail as well.

4. Tell the examiner which colleagues you would call to support you (e.g. critical care outreach, trauma doctors, A+E consultant).

The above examples of scenarios therefore become:

- A+E calls you to see a 12-year-old boy with a short history of testicular pain.

   "I recognise this as a potential urological emergency as this patient sounds like he might have a testicular torsion (1). I will therefore see him myself without delay (2). On arrival I will introduce myself and undertake a rapid systematic A-to-E assessment (3). Provided his observations are within normal range, I would proceed to take a focused urological history with a paediatric nurse present (4)".

- The ward calls you about your patient, on whom you performed a TURP this afternoon, informing you that he is drowsy, febrile and his blood pressure is low.

   "I recognise this as a potential urological emergency as this patient sounds like he might be suffering with post-operative urinary sepsis (1). I will therefore see him myself without delay (2). On arrival I will introduce myself and undertake a rapid systematic A-to-E assessment following the CCrISP algorithm and because there has been a documented fever, I will complete the Sepsis-6 bundle (3) and inform critical care outreach about this patient (4). Provided his observations are within normal range, I would proceed to take a focused urological history".

To a degree it will depend on the type of patient you are presented with, but the points I am trying to drive home are:

A. Make it clear that you recognise it is urgent and state what your primary concern is.

B. Always undertake some form of A-to-E assessment, even if brief or simply a mention, as omission of this may cost you marks but a mention will protect you against all eventualities. Be prepared to potentially expand on the individual A-to-E components if asked and throw in the Sepsis-6 bundle if there is a mere whiff of potential sepsis.

C. Be pro-active and take charge, but do not work alone i.e. involve your colleague consultant intensivist, microbiologist etc.

DISCUSSING SCANS/IMAGES

During your FRCS (Urol) Section 2 viva exam, it is a guarantee that you will be given a scan, image or visual resource to discuss and interpret.

This may even be the first question you get at the start of the station to lead you into the scenario, or the image could be handed to you after you have "assessed" a patient and stated that you would request further imaging as part of your management plan.

Scans/images realistically can pertain to anything within the FRCS (Urol) syllabus; however, a non-exhaustive common list of images that may be given to you include:

- Imaging: CT KUB/urogram/abdomen, MRI prostate, US urinary tract, NM bone scan, plain XRs

- Devices: stents, baskets

- Photos of lithotripter machines, imaging machines (CT scanners, US probes etc.)

- Urodynamic traces (covered in the urodynamics section).

Candidates often panic when handed an image to interpret – and understandably so, as the clock is ticking in the background and the expectation is that you will be able to know what it is and spot all the relevant findings quickly. Truth be told, if you really have no clue what it is then it will be a challenge and you will lose marks for prompting by the examiners; however, with meticulous and broad practice you will have seen most types of images that may arise before and you will be fine.

As ever, having a structure for these answers is fundamental for many reasons. It will allow you to begin your answer without undue pauses, you will appear structured and organised, and it will also help you inadvertently spot things that you might otherwise have missed. Above all when you follow a structure and observe another candidate using it in a simulation viva, you will appreciate the true power and efficacy of it, which ultimately translates into more marks in your exam.

Patient Scan Images

For all patient scan images that are shown to you, I recommend you use the following structure when answering a request to *"Describe what you see on this scan"*.

1. Tell the examiner <u>what type of imaging modality and body part</u> it is and state that you would confirm that it pertains to the patient in question, for example:

   - *"This is a non-contrast CT KUB, which I would confirm pertains to the patient in question"* (A)

   - *"This is a grey-scale US single image of a bladder, which I would confirm pertains to the patient in question"* (B).

(With CT urinary tract scans, try to identify whether it is with or without contrast by looking for white contrast in the bladder or ureters. If you really are not sure, cover yourself by saying *"I am looking for contrast in the urinary tract but cannot confidently see any"*.)

2. Tell the examiner <u>what is the most obvious/striking abnormality</u> first, for example:

   - *"The most striking abnormality I can see is a large stone filling most of the renal pelvis in the patient's left kidney"* (A)

   - *"The most striking abnormality I can see is a large papillary mass on the patient's left wall of the bladder which concerns me for a bladder tumour* (B).

3. Tell the examiner what other <u>relevant positive</u> findings (if any) you can see, for example using (A) and (B) above:

   - *"I can also see another small stone in the lower pole of the same kidney"* (A)

   - *"I can also see a urinary catheter in situ"*. (B)

4. Tell the examiner what <u>relevant negative</u> findings you are looking for but cannot find, for example using (A) and (B) above:

   - *"I am looking for stones in the ureter and contra-lateral kidney, signs of cortical atrophy or scarring, but I cannot see any on this single image"* (A)

   - *"I am looking for evidence of metachronous bladder tumours, enlarged lymph nodes and features of metastatic disease, but I cannot see any on this single image"*. (B)

You have to apply a degree of common sense and knowledge when proposing relevant negatives.

For example a CT scan showing an "unhappy" kidney in a septic patient should raise the suspicion of emphysematous pyelonephritis or renal abscess as potential differential diagnoses; therefore, even if you have not seen any such features to suggest these, you should comment:

e.g. *"I am looking for gas or collections in the kidney which would suggest emphysematous pyelonephritis or renal abscess, but cannot see any"*.

Try to be open minded about what other differential diagnoses the scan could represent (e.g. a swelling in a kidney on US could arguably be a stone, small angiomyolipoma or complex cyst), and therefore in turn propose a radiological finding you are looking for to evaluate these alternatives but subsequently refute them:

e.g. *"I cannot see any acoustic shadow behind this swelling which suggests it is not a stone"*.

5. Tell the examiner what is your <u>final conclusion/diagnosis</u> based on your interpretation of the image, for example using (A) and (B) above:

    •   *"In conclusion based on this CT scan, this patient has a large staghorn calculus in the left kidney" (A)*

    •   *"In conclusion based on this US scan, this patient has a single large bladder tumour on the left side". (B)*

6. Tell the examiner the <u>standard closing phrase</u>:

    •   *"I would wish to see the full complement of images that complete the series, verifying my findings by checking the full radiology report and discussing these with my colleague consultant uro-radiologist".*

That way, even if you have potentially missed something, arguably you have played safe by cross-checking the scan with a radiologist.

Machines/Devices/Objects

You may get a photo of an imaging machine (e.g. CT scanner) or of an object (e.g. ureteric stent or basket). Questions about these are likely to revolve around:

•   What is this?

•   What is it made of/what are the components of this setup?

•   How does it work?

If you have thoroughly revised your urological technology section, answering these questions should be straightforward. If, however, you are weak in technology knowledge, you will really struggle to survive a station featuring a series of photos of objects and urological devices.

Try to prepare a ready-made memorised two- or three-sentence statement which you can state confidently for what each imaging modality is and how it works (i.e. US, CT, MR, nuclear medicine, XR). This will at least allow you to cruise on a 6 (pass) whilst you try to gain marks elsewhere.

CONSENTING PATIENTS

It is almost certain that at some point in the exam you will be asked to describe how you would consent a patient for a particular urology procedure. As it is a consultant exam after all, you should realistically be able to consent a patient for any procedure that is performed in a standard DGH urology department.

Again I invite you to practise using a structure to answer this question. The one I used is simple and we use it in our everyday job – namely to follow the sections of a standard consent form of the kind we ask patients to sign in our UK hospitals. For example:

Describe how you would consent this patient for right-sided PCNL.

1. Start with the full (i.e. not abbreviated) name of the procedure:

    *   *"I would inform the patient that we are proposing to list them for a right-sided* <u>percutaneous nephro-lithotomy</u>*".*

2. State the <u>benefits/reason for</u> doing this operation:

    *   *"I would tell them we are doing this operation with the aim of treating and clearing the stone in their right kidney, which will help their symptoms".*

3. State the <u>risks of</u> doing this operation:

    *   *"More common risks of this operation include pain, infection, minor bleeding, further stone formation in the future; less common risks include severe bleeding requiring embolisation (1 in 100), bowel injury, and very rarely bleeding requiring emergency nephrectomy (less than 1 in a 1,000)".*

I have chosen to structure my complications as "more common", "less common" or "rare" as I always think common things are common, and by using this strategy you will sound in turn like someone with common sense.

You could alternatively choose to categorise your risks using "immediate", "early" and "late" or "mild", "moderate" and "severe" – provided you are structured with your answer, I am sure this would also be fine.

You are not expected to be exhaustive, with an endless list of possible complications; however, a well-structured answer which flows sensibly, mentioning the key ones (there are always exam favourites such 1% risk of embolisation in PCNL or 5–7% risk of positive margin in partial nephrectomy) will ensure you sail through this answer.

I strongly recommend that for each operation, you look at the relevant BAUS information leaflet. The leaflets helpfully list the risks in order of descending chance of these happening, which really helps you structure your answer.

4.   State the <u>alternatives</u> to doing this operation:

   • *"I would explain that potential alternatives to this operation include conservative management or staged ureteroscopy + LASER surgeries".*

5.   Conclude by saying:

   • *"I would sign and date the consent form myself and offer the patient the opportunity to sign themselves if they are in agreement".*

Finally, you may be asked about the Montgomery principle of informed consent, so it is worth briefly outlining this here.

Prior to Montgomery, the doctor's duty to counsel patients of risks was based on whether they had acted in line with a responsible body of medical opinion. Put simply, you could detail the same standard list of risks to all patients undergoing the same procedure, regardless of who the patient was.

Following Montgomery, doctors must inform about all material risks as well as disclosing any risk to which a reasonable person in the patient's position would attach significance. In other words, doctors must discuss the standard list of risks as above, <u>plus</u> any to which it would be reasonable for them to think the <u>individual</u> patient would attach particular significance.

It goes without saying, therefore, that current practices of pooled lists operating on patients you have never met, on-the-day consenting after prolonged waiting times etc. all make adhering to Montgomery consent very challenging indeed.

TROUBLESHOOTING

The Section 2 viva is an exam covering a wide breadth of knowledge and the stations are delivered at pace with many questions, therefore it is likely that at some point you might not know the answer to a particular question and nerves might not help either.

Fear not – passing or failing does not hinge on a single question.

Indeed not knowing an answer but proposing a sensible, safe strategy to mitigate the gap in your knowledge may settle you on a safe 6 (pass) anyway – provided you haven't got gaps in your knowledge for all the other questions in the station, of course!

Whilst I do not suggest bringing politics into the exam, politicians can be astute in dealing with questions they do not know how to answer, so it might be worth taking a leaf out of their books. For example, it is preferable to say *"I am sorry, I cannot recall the answer"* (which is polite and suggests you knew it but have temporarily forgotten) as opposed to *"I don't know"* (which implies you never knew or read about this in the first place and furthermore aren't sorry).

As ever, I recommend practising the simple techniques of self-defence that I have detailed below to protect you in the eventuality that you do not know an answer. This list is far from exhaustive but should get you thinking further about how to deal with potential blank moments.

Questions about Drugs/Medicines

If you do not know the answer about a drug dosage, options include:

- *"I would check this in the latest edition of the BNF"*
- *"I would contact my Trust on-call pharmacist to discuss this"*.

If you do not know the answer about a particular choice of antibiotics, options include:

- *"I would consult the antibiotic guidelines on my Trust intranet page to safeguard my antibiotic stewardship practice"*
- *"I would personally contact my consultant colleague on-call microbiologist"*.

Questions about Scans

If you cannot interpret a scan that you have been given then admittedly it will be difficult to get the scenario flowing without prompting; however, just to remain calm and say something sensible, you may state:

- *"I am not sure what this scan shows, but I would personally discuss this with my on-call colleague uro-radiologist to see if they can guide me further (urgent scenario)"*
- *"I am not sure what this scan shows, but I would personally discuss this at my departmental benign x-ray meeting with my trusted uro-radiologist present to see if they can guide me further" (elective scenario).*

Questions about Sub-specialised Interventions

As a day-one consultant urologist in a DGH, you would not realistically be expected to perform a neobladder formation or bladder augmentation independently, so if you are asked how you would do this operation it is safe to say:

- *"I would ensure that my senior consultant colleague specialist in pelvic oncology/reconstruction is present during my operating list for dual consultant operating".*

Be careful not to say this for those operations you would be expected to perform (e.g. TURP, PCNL) otherwise you will appear lacking in confidence and not ready to achieve completion of training in urology.

ANSWERS TO MCQS

Station 5: Calculi & Urinary Tract Infections

1. D
2. B
3. C
4. A
5. A
6. E
7. A
8. B
9. B
10. D
11. C
12. E
13. D
14. C
15. A
16. B
17. E
18. E
19. C
20. D

Station 6: Urological Imaging & Principles of Urological Technology

1. B
2. B
3. B
4. D
5. A
6. E

7. C

8. C

9. D

10. C

11. C

12. B

13. E

14. E

15. E

16. A

17. D

18. A

19. C

20. B

Station 7: Bladder Dysfunction & Gynaecological Aspects of Urology

1. A

2. A

3. C

4. E

5. B

6. D

7. C

8. D

9. A

10. D

11. E

12. B – the AMS 600 is a penile malleable prosthesis

13. D

14. B

15. C

16. C

17. A

18. C

19. E

20. B

Station 8: Andrology & BPH

1. D – the other medications are unlicensed indications

2. B

3. A

4. B

5. E – it is $< 10^5$; however, the samples have to be minimum 4 weeks apart, so 14 weeks would be too soon for special clearance to be given

6. C

7. D

8. D

9. E

10. B

11. A

12. B

13. C

14. E – the correct answer is 4%

15. A

16. E – the correct answer is IFN-α2b

17. C

18. D – figures are from Abrams 1979

19. B

20. B – figures are from Abrams 1979

21. C

22. A

23. E – correct answer is tamsulosin vs. dutasteride vs. combination therapy

24. D

25. A

ADDITIONAL MCQS

STATION 5: CALCULI & URINARY TRACT INFECTIONS MCQS

1. Which of the following does not increase your risk of stone formation in urinary tract?

    A) Roux-en-Y gastric bypass
    B) High calcium intake
    C) Testosterone supplementation
    D) Horseshoe kidney
    E) Corticosteroids

2. Which of the following is the best description of the shape appearance of uric acid stones under light microscopy?

    A) Pyramidal
    B) Coffin lids
    C) Hexagonal
    D) Rectangular
    E) Dumbbell

3. Which of the following is the correct range of attenuation values (HU) for uric acid stones?

    A) 200–400
    B) 400–600
    C) 600–800
    D) 800–1,000
    E) 1,000–1,400

4. Which of the following statements regarding the SUSPEND trial is false?

    A) Albeit not achieving statistical significance, the nifedipine group had marginally fewer patients requiring treatment within 4 weeks
    B) Adherence to medication was not assessed
    C) Patients with GFR < 30mL/minute were excluded
    D) Primary outcome was need for stone clearance treatment within 4 weeks of entry
    E) Patients were randomised to tamsulosin vs. nifedipine vs. placebo (1:1:1)

5. *Regarding complete ureteral occlusion, which of the following statements is true?*

   A) After 60 minutes there is decreased renal blood flow
   B) After 60 minutes there is no change in renal blood flow
   C) After 90 minutes there is post-glomerular vasoconstriction
   D) After 90 minutes there is post-glomerular vasodilatation
   E) None of the above

6. *Which one of the following is not an amino acid whose transport defect is associated with homozygous cystinuria?*

   A) Lysine
   B) Cysteine
   C) Arginine
   D) Ornithine
   E) All of the above

7. *A patient undergoing investigations for prostatitis, has completed a Meares and Stamey four glass test. VB1 and VB2 have cultured negative, however VB3 culture reveals white cells. Which type of prostatitis as per NIDDK classification does this patient have?*

   A) I
   B) II
   C) IIIA
   D) IIIB
   E) IV

8. *Which of these antibiotics works by inhibiting DNA gyrase?*

   A) Ciprofloxacin
   B) Doxycycline
   C) Nitrofurantoin
   D) Cefalexin
   E) Tazobactam

9. Which of the following statements regarding the diagnosis of urethritis is correct?

   A) Requires ≥ 20 polymorph nuclear leucocytes / HPF from urethral smear

   B) Requires ≥ 50 polymorph nuclear leucocytes / HPF from urethral smear

   C) Requires ≥ 100 polymorph nuclear leucocytes / HPF from urethral smear

   D) Requires ≥ 5 polymorph nuclear leucocytes / HPF from first voided urine

   E) Requires ≥ 10 polymorph nuclear leucocytes / HPF from first voided urine

10. Which of the following statements regarding bilharzia is incorrect?

    A) Skin penetration occurs by cercariae

    B) Areas endemic with s.japonicum have higher rates of seizures than baseline

    C) Belongs to group of helminth infections

    D) Ureteric involvement is normally to the distal ureter

    E) The name of the intermediate host snail for S.mansoni is bulinus

11. Which of the statements regarding urinary TB is incorrect?

    A) Gram-positive organisms stain violet

    B) Lowenstein–Jensen culture takes ≥ 6 weeks

    C) Spread to bladder features a yellow lesion with red halo

    D) Pyrazinamide may cause peripheral neuropathy

    E) Epididymal involvement is usually unilateral

12. What is the sheath size used in ultra-mini PCNL?

    A) 4.5–6F
    B) 7–10F
    C) 11–13F
    D) 14–16F
    E) 17–20F

13. Regarding the holmium:YAG LASER, the zone of thermal injury from LASER tip is limited to:

    A) 0–0.5mm
    B) 0–1.0mm
    C) 0–2.5mm
    D) 0–5.0mm
    E) 0–10mm

14. Which crystal shape best describes those of weddellite stones seen under light microscopy?

    A) Pyramidal
    B) Hexagonal
    C) Rectangular
    D) Dumbell
    E) Coffin lid

15. Which of the following is an inhibitor of stone formation?

    A) Pyrophosphate
    B) Sodium phosphate
    C) Magnesium phosphate
    D) Potassium phosphate
    E) Orthophosphate

16. Which of the following regarding renal leak hypercalciuria is false?

    A) Urinary calcium loss occurs regardless of serum calcium levels
    B) Urinary calcium loss is unaffected by dietary calcium
    C) Serum PTH is raised
    D) It is associated with multicystic dysplastic kidney
    E) Serum calcium is raised

17. Which of the following regarding staghorn calculi is false?

    A) Staphylococcus heterogeneously produces urease
    B) They are more common in women
    C) Mycoplasma is a urea-splitting organism
    D) Acetohydraxamic acid is a direct antagonist of urease
    E) The crystal shape under light microscopy is coffin lid

18. Which of the following statements regarding urolithiasis and hydronephrosis in pregnancy is false?

    A) Pregnant women have a higher excretion of magnesium vs. non-pregnant women
    B) Pregnant women have a higher excretion of uric acid vs. non-pregnant women
    C) Progesterone promotes ureteric smooth dilatation
    D) Non-urgent URS is best performed in 2nd rather than 1st trimester
    E) Nitrofurantoin avoided due to potential teratogenicity on foetal neurodevelopment

19. *Which of the following statements regarding cystinuria is false?*

    A) Homozygous and heterozygous cystinuria have no difference in phenotype
    B) Brand's test relies on cyanide converting cystine to cysteine
    C) Penicillamine can be used as an oral chelator of cystine
    D) Crystals appear hexagonal under white light microscopy
    E) α-MPG is an oral chelator of cystine

20. *What substance on a standard urine dipstick comes into contact with haemoglobin, which leads to an oxidation reaction and cell lysis?*

    A) Tetrabromophenol
    B) Orthotolidine
    C) Indoxyl
    D) Diazonium chromogen
    E) Sodium nitroprusside

21. *Which chemical found in cranberry juice is thought to be responsible for its action in preventing rUTI in women?*

    A) Seminose
    B) Proanthocyanidin
    C) GAG
    D) Sodium hyaluronate
    E) u.ursi

22. *Which of the following statements regarding mumps orchitis is true?*

    A) Seminiferous tubule necrosis occurs by pressure
    B) Orchitis is more common in pre- rather than post-pubertal males
    C) The incubation period is 5–7 days
    D) Mumps is a RNA adenovirus disease
    E) It causes oligospermia/azoospermia, but not asthenospermia

23. *Which of the following best fits the description of category IV prostatitis?*

    A) Inflammatory CPPS
    B) Chronic bacterial prostatitis
    C) Chronic abacterial prostatitis
    D) Asymptomatic inflammatory prostatitis
    E) Non-inflammatory CPPS

24. *Which cell type is characteristically found in XGP?*

    A) Acrophage
    B) Polymorphonuclear cell
    C) Lipid laden macrophage
    D) Giant cell
    E) NK cell

25. *Chlamydia trachomatis is:*

    A) Not a holoparasite
    B) Facultative parasite
    C) Gram-positive rod
    D) Gram-positive coccus
    E) Gram-negative coccus

STATION 6: UROLOGICAL IMAGING & PRINCIPLES OF UROLOGICAL TECHNOLOGY MCQS

1. Which of the following sutures is not absorbable?

    A) Monocryl
    B) Vicryl
    C) Catgut
    D) Polypropylene
    E) Polydioxanone

2. How many times per hour is the air changed in the operating theatre in conventional ventilation systems?

    A) 20–40
    B) 40–60
    C) 60–80
    D) 80–100
    E) 100–120

3. What is the correct wavelength (nm) for KTP Greenlight LASER?

    A) 266
    B) 532
    C) 1,064
    D) 2,013
    E) 2,140

4. What is the penetration depth (mm) of the Ho:YAG LASER?

    A) 0.1
    B) 0.2
    C) 0.4
    D) 0.8
    E) 10

5. What is the correct diameter (inches) for a typical guidewire in endourology?

    A) 0.035
    B) 0.048
    C) 0.125
    D) 0.148
    E) 0.152

6. Which parameter is not included as part of the MDRD formula for calculating GFR?

    A) Age
    B) Gender
    C) Serum creatinine
    D) Ethnicity
    E) Body mass

7. What is the approximate half-life of 99mTc?

    A) 24 hours
    B) 18 hours
    C) 12 hours
    D) 9 hours
    E) 6 hours

8. Which radioisotope does the PMSA scan use?

    A) 11C
    B) 68Ga
    C) 131I
    D) 99mTc
    E) 192Ir

9. What is the correct external diameter (mm) of a 24Fr cystoscope?

    A) 24
    B) 16
    C) 12
    D) 8
    E) 6

10. The nursing assistant passes you a cystoscope with a red label. What is the correct degree angle of this scope?

    A) 0
    B) 12
    C) 30
    D) 70
    E) None of the above

11. *Ureteric stents are radiopaque – which metal/alloy do they contain which allows for this property?*

    A) Bismuth
    B) Iron
    C) Steel
    D) Nickel
    E) Titanium

12. *What gauge (Fr) is a urinary catheter with an orange-coloured label?*

    A) 12
    B) 14
    C) 16
    D) 18
    E) 20

13. *Which of the following is not a recognised stage of biofilm formation?*

    A) Aggregation
    B) Adhesion
    C) 3D growth
    D) Replication
    E) Microorganism release

14. *During ESWL, what is the approximate pressure value at the top of positive phase waveform of the acoustic shockwave?*

    A) 10MPa
    B) 40Mpa
    C) 10KPa
    D) 40KPa
    E) 80Kpa

15. *What type of energy does the harmonic scalpel use?*

    A) Monopolar
    B) Bipolar
    C) Thermal
    D) Radiofrequency
    E) Ultrasound

16. *What level of evidence is a well-designed, controlled experimental study?*

    A) 1a
    B) 1b
    C) 2a
    D) 2b
    E) 3

17. *What is the correct osmolarity (mOsm/L) for 1.5% glycine solution?*

    A) 200
    B) 220
    C) 230
    D) 250
    E) 280

18. *What type of energy does the ligasure device use?*

    A) Monopolar
    B) Bipolar
    C) Thermal
    D) Radiofrequency
    E) Ultrasound

19. *What are LASER fibres made of?*

    A) Nitinol
    B) Silica
    C) PTFE
    D) Carbon
    E) Titanium

20. *What is the correct wavelength (nm) for Ho:YAG LASER?*

    A) 266
    B) 532
    C) 1,064
    D) 2,013
    E) 2,140

STATION 7: BLADDER DYSFUNCTION & GYNAECOLOGICAL ASPECTS OF UROLOGY MCQS

1. *Where do the fibres of the pudendal nerve originate from?*
   A) Ventromedial nucleus
   B) Barrington's nucleus
   C) Onuf's nucleus
   D) Clarke's nucleus
   E) Periaqueductal grey

2. *Below which spinal level is autonomic dysreflexia less likely to occur?*
   A) T4
   B) T6
   C) T8
   D) T10
   E) T12

3. *What is the correct minimum PFMT regime as recommended by NICE (2019)?*
   A) ≥ 6 contractions, twice daily
   B) ≥ 8 contractions, twice daily
   C) ≥ 4 contractions, three times daily
   D) ≥ 6 contractions, three times daily
   E) ≥ 8 contractions, three times daily

4. *Which of the following is not a contraindication to anticholinergic medication?*
   A) Congestive heart failure
   B) Pyloric stenosis
   C) Severe ulcerative colitis
   D) Urinary retention
   E) Intestinal atony

5. *Which muscarinic receptors does tolterodine primarily block?*
   A) M1
   B) M2
   C) M3
   D) M2 and M3
   E) None of the above

6. What is the approximate half-life of solifenacin?

    A) 15–30 hours
    B) 30–45 hours
    C) 45–60 hours
    D) 60–75 hours
    E) 75–90 hours

7. What is the approximate half-life of mirabegron?

    A) 10 hours
    B) 20 hours
    C) 30 hours
    D) 40 hours
    E) 50 hours

8. Which statement regarding the DIGNITY study for BOTOX is false?

    A) The trigone was not injected
    B) Both MS and SCI patients benefited
    C) Only neuropathic patients were included
    D) No difference in efficacy was noted between 100units and 200units dose
    E) The end-point follow up was after 6 weeks

9. If VLPP is noted to be < 60cm H_2O during UDS assessment for SUI, what is the most likely underlying problem?

    A) Detrusor hyperreflexia
    B) Anatomical cause
    C) Urethral hypermobility
    D) Hypotonic detrusor muscle
    E) Intrinsic sphincter deficiency

10. Which of the following statements regarding duloxetine is false?

    A) Inhibits reuptake of noradrenaline
    B) It can be prescribed for a patient also taking warfarin
    C) Yawning is a common side-effect
    D) Severe diarrhoea and vomiting should prompt immediate cessation
    E) It can be prescribed in pregnancy

11. *What pressure should the pressure-regulating balloon be set at in the AUS device?*

    A) 41–50cm H_2O
    B) 51–60cm H_2O
    C) 61–70cm H_2O
    D) 71–80cm H_2O
    E) 81–90cm H_2O

12. *A patient who has undergone UDS has a Qmax of 12mL/s and PdetQmax of 77cm H_2O. What is the correct value of their bladder outlet obstruction index?*

    A) 53
    B) 41
    C) 89
    D) 101
    E) 65

13. *What is the approximate adherence rate after 12 months for patients starting anticholinergic medication?*

    A) 20–25%
    B) 30–35%
    C) 40–45%
    D) 50–55%
    E) 60–65%

14. *Which statement is correct regarding the motor innervation of the bladder is true?*

    A) Post-ganglionic parasympathetic nuclei are located at S2–4
    B) The predominant effect of the sympathetic nerves is parasympathetic inhibition
    C) Parasympathetic nerves provide cholinergic inhibitory input to the detrusor
    D) Parasympathetic nerves provide excitatory input to the bladder neck
    E) The nuclei of the pre-ganglionic sympathetic nerves lie in the hypogastric plexus

15. A patient who has undergone UDS has a Qmax of 12mL/s and PdetQmax of 77cm H_2O. What is the correct value of their bladder contractility index?

    A) 17
    B) 101
    C) 137
    D) 113
    E) 41

16. Which nerve roots does the bulbocavernous reflex test?

    A) T10 – S2
    B) T12 – S2
    C) T12 – S4
    D) S2 – S4
    E) S1 – S2

17. Which of the following statements regarding the urethral sphincter innervation is false?

    A) Perineal branch of pudendal nerve is for motor input
    B) Relaxation is mediated by nitric oxide
    C) Onuf's nucleus is located in the ventral part of the anterior horn of the sacral cord
    D) The intrinsic sphincter is absent anteriorly
    E) The skeletal muscle component is the outermost layer

18. Where is the periaqueductal grey matter located?

    A) Within tegmentum of midbrain
    B) Within corpora quadrigemina around the cerebral aqueduct
    C) Within the substancia nigra
    D) Within the reticular formation
    E) Within the crus cerebri

19. Which of the following statements regarding mirabegron is true?

    A) It inhibits adenylyl cyclase
    B) It is metabolised by the kidneys and excreted in the urine
    C) Angioedema is a common side-effect
    D) It is safe in breast feeding
    E) It promotes cAMP stimulation

20. *What is the most common type of cancer found in female urethral diverticulum?*

    A) Transitional cell carcinoma
    B) Adenocarcinoma
    C) Squamous cell carcinoma
    D) Sarcoma
    E) Mucinous cell carcinoma

STATION 8: ANDROLOGY & BPH MCQS

1. *Which of the following statements is correct?*

    A) Dutasteride inhibits type-1 5AR enzyme only
    B) Dutasteride inhibits both type-1 and type-2 5AR enzymes
    C) Finasteride inhibits type-1 5AR enzyme only
    D) Finasteride inhibits type-1 and type-2 5AR enzymes
    E) None of the above

2. *Which medication can cause retrograde ejaculation as a side-effect?*

    A) Chloral hydrate
    B) Chlorambucil
    C) Chlordiazepoxide
    D) Chlorpromazine
    E) None of the above

3. *Testosterone supplementation may cause one of the following:*

    A) Basophilia
    B) Eosinophilia
    C) Rise in haematocrit
    D) Thrombocytopenia
    E) None of the above

4. *Which of the following statements is correct?*

    A) LH decreases cholesterol desmolase activity
    B) Prolactin decreases the response of Leydig cells to LH
    C) Leydig cells are polyhedral in shape
    D) Testosterone provides positive feedback to the hypothalamus
    E) None of the above

5. *Which of the following statements regarding Peyronie's disease is incorrect?*

    A) It is more common in Caucasian rather than Afro-Caribbean men
    B) Typical age of onset is 60–70 years
    C) Penile ultrasonography typically reveals hyperechoic thickened tunica albuginea
    D) It is associated with Ledderhose disease
    E) Tamoxifen modulates fibroblast secretion and thus more effective in acute phase

6. Which of the following is not a recognised side-effect of tamsulosin?

    A) Papillitis
    B) Asthenia
    C) Stevens–Johnson syndrome
    D) Angioedema
    E) Diarrhoea

7. Which of the following is not a recognised risk factor for developing AUR?

    A) IPSS > 5
    B) PSA > 1.4
    C) Qmax < 12mL/s
    D) Age > 70 years
    E) Prostate volume > 30mL

8. Which phytotherapy agent has not been used to treat BPH symptoms?

    A) Pygeum africanum
    B) Saw palmetto
    C) Beta-sitosterol
    D) Secale cereale
    E) Ferula persica

9. Regarding surgical treatment for Peyronie's disease, which of the following statements is true?

    A) The most commonly used autograft for the Lue procedure is the saphenous vein
    B) Lue procedure has a lower risk of ED than Nesbit plication
    C) Yachia procedure is a form of concave lengthening procedure
    D) 75% of patients undergoing Nesbit's procedure will require a circumcision
    E) Residual penile curvature < 20° after plication is uncommon in high-volume centres

10. An isolated deficiency in LH is found in which condition?

    A) Kallman syndrome
    B) Leydig cell hypoplasia
    C) Swyer syndrome
    D) Pasqualini syndrome
    E) Jacob's syndrome

11. *Which one of the following lower reference limit values as per WHO (2010) semen analysis parameters is incorrect?*

    A) Sperm morphology > 4% normal forms
    B) Total sperm count > 39 x 10^6
    C) Sperm concentration > 12 x 10^6/mL
    D) Semen volume > 1.5 mL
    E) Progressive motility > 32%

12. *Which of the following is not a symptom that features on the IPSS questionnaire?*

    A) Straining
    B) Intermittency
    C) Urgency
    D) Incomplete emptying
    E) Hesitancy

13. *Which of the following is not a recognised side-effect of sildenafil?*

    A) Gynaecomastia
    B) Oculogyric crisis
    C) Myalgia
    D) Insomnia
    E) Scleral discoloration

14. *What approximate proportion of patients treated with PDE5i drugs do not respond?*

    A) 5%
    B) 10%
    C) 20%
    D) 30%
    E) 40%

15. *The CONDUCT study for BPH evaluated the following medication against watchful waiting:*

    A) Dutasteride and alfuzosin
    B) Dutasteride and terazosin
    C) Finasteride and alfuzosin
    D) Finasteride and terazosin
    E) None of the above

16. *Which artery does the common penile artery arise from?*

    A) Internal pudendal artery
    B) Anterior branch of internal iliac artery
    C) Posterior branch of internal iliac artery
    D) External pudendal artery
    E) Superficial external pudendal artery

17. *Where is the somatic centre for efferent innervation of ischio- and bulbocavernous muscles of the penis?*

    A) Onuf's nucleus
    B) Marginal nucleus
    C) Nucleus propius
    D) Nucleus solitarius
    E) Edinger–Westphal nucleus

18. *What proportion of circulating testosterone is free?*

    A) < 1%
    B) 2%
    C) 5%
    D) 10%
    E) 20%

19. *The precursor to the primary spermatocyte is:*

    A) Preleptotene spermatocyte
    B) Intermediate spermatogonium
    C) Spermatid
    D) Type-A spermatogonium
    E) Type-B spermatogonium

20. *Globozoospermia is best defined as:*

    A) Increase in viscosity of sperm
    B) High percentage of immotile sperm
    C) Sperm lacking acrosomal caps
    D) High percentage of dead sperm
    E) Sperm heads are tapered

21. *The mechanism of action of POTABA to treat Peyronie's disease is best described as:*

A) Inhibits collagen by increasing serotonin levels
B) Activates free radicals to reduce oxidative stress
C) Inactivates free radicals to reduce oxidative stress
D) Increases serotonin levels to decrease fibrosis
E) Decreases serotonin levels to decrease fibrosis

22. *What is the average half-life of unbound testosterone?*

A) 24–48 hours
B) ≤ 24 hours
C) ≤ 6 hours
D) 10–15 minutes
E) < 5 minutes

23. *Which of the following statements regarding UroLift™ is true?*

A) MRI is safe provided the static magnetic field is of ≤ 3 Tesla
B) MRI is safe provided the static magnetic field is of ≤ 5 Tesla
C) Patients with UroLift™ should not have an MRI scan
D) It is safe in all MRI scanners
E) None of the above

24. *Which of the following criteria does not feature on the IIEF-5 questionnaire for ED?*

A) Patient difficulty in maintaining an erection after penetration
B) Patient frequency of achieving erection adequate for penetration
C) Patient difficulty in maintaining an erection to complete intercourse
D) Patient perceived rigidity of erection
E) Patient frequency of satisfaction in sexual intercourse

25. *What is the half-life of tadalafil?*

A) ~ 24 hours
B) ~ 17 hours
C) ~ 13 hours
D) ~ 9 hours
E) ~ 6 hours

26. *Which of the following statements regarding Doppler study of penile blood flow in erection for EDC assessment is true?*

    A) End diastolic velocity is normal if > 10cm/s
    B) End diastolic velocity is normal if > 5cm/s
    C) Peak systolic velocity is abnormal if < 25cm/s
    D) Peak systolic velocity is abnormal if < 35cm/s
    E) None of the above

27. *Which of the following groups of IIEF-5 questionnaire scores is correct as per the different categories of ED severity?*

    A) 1–6, 7–10, 11–15, 16–21, 22–25
    B) 1–7, 8–11, 12–16, 17–21, 22–25
    C) 1–5, 6–10, 11–16, 17–21, 22–25
    D) 1–7, 8–12, 13–17, 18–21, 22–25
    E) 1–6, 7–10, 11–15, 16–20, 21–25

28. *What is the correct late failure rate for vasectomy?*

    A) 1 in 500
    B) 1 in 1,000
    C) 1 in 1,500
    D) 1 in 2,000
    E) 1 in 2,500

29. *All of the following are contraindications to PDE5i use except:*

    A) Active peptic ulceration
    B) Hereditary degenerative retinal disorder
    C) History of non-arteritic anterior ischaemic optic neuropathy
    D) Recent history of antero-lateral myocardial infarction
    E) Recent history of postero-lateral myocardial infarction

30. *Which of the following statements about PDE5i drugs is true?*

    A) They convert ATP to cAMP
    B) They convert GTP to GMP
    C) They convert GMP to cGMP
    D) They convert GTP to cGMP
    E) They convert cGMP to GMP

ANSWERS TO ADDITIONAL MCQS

STATION 5: CALCULI & URINARY TRACT INFECTIONS

1. B – low calcium intake is correct

2. D

3. A

4. A

5. C

6. B – cysteine should be "cystine" (cystine is oxidised dimer form of cysteine)

7. C

8. A

9. E

10. E – bulinus is the intermediate snail host for S.haematobium, not S.mansoni (the name of the intermediate host is biomphalaria)

11. D – isoniazid may cause peripheral neuropathy

12. C

13. B

14. A – weddellite is calcium oxalate dihydrate

15. A

16. D – renal leak hypercalciuria is associated with medullary sponge kidney

17. D – acetohydraamic acid is a competitive inhibitor of urease (its molecule is similar to urea but not hydrolysable by urease), pH ≥ 7.2 favours staghorn formation

18. E – nitrofurantoin is potentially harmful in pregnancy as may cause haemolytic anaemia

19. C – penicillamine binds to cysteine

20. B

21. B

22. A – mumps is an RNA paramyxovirus disease

23. D

24. C

25. E – chlamydia is a Gram-negative coccus, but it is also an obligate parasite (i.e. cannot complete life cycle without host exploitation); holoparasite is another term for obligate parasite

STATION 6: UROLOGICAL IMAGING & PRINCIPLES OF UROLOGICAL TECHNOLOGY

1. D – polypropylene is prolene, which is non-absorbable

2. A

3. B

4. C

5. A

6. E

7. E

8. B

9. D – recall the diameter corresponds to a 1/3 of the French gauge

10. C

11. A

12. C

13. D

14. B

15. E

16. C

17. A

18. B

19. B

20. E

STATION 7: BLADDER DYSFUNCTION & GYNAECOLOGICAL ASPECTS OF UROLOGY

1. C

2. B

3. E

4. A – heart failure is a caution, not a contraindication

5. E

6. C

7. E

8. D – note the doses given were 200units and 300units (neuropaths are usually offered a higher starting dose compared to patients with IDO)

9. E

10. D – in this case duloxetine should be stopped; however, it is recommended always to taper down the dose over 1–2 weeks

11. C

12. A

13. B

14. B

15. C

16. D

17. D – the intrinsic sphincter is absent posteriorly

18. A

19. E – angioedema is rare; it is metabolised by the liver but indeed excreted in the urine

20. B

STATION 8: ANDROLOGY & BPH

1. B

2. D – chlorpromazine is an anti-psychotic drug which also possesses antiserotonergic properties.

3. C – the haematocrit should be checked at baseline and yearly if testosterone treatment ongoing

4. C

5. B – Peyronie's is most common in men aged 50–60 years

6. A

7. A – IPSS > 7 is a recognised risk factor for developing AUR in men

8. E

9. A – note that circumcision required in 25%, and minor residual curvature is common

10. D

11. C – sperm concentration $> 15 \times 10^6$/mL (WHO semen analysis parameters are an exam favourite, and these should be memorised confidently)

12. E

13. B

14. D

15. E – CONDUCT study evaluated dutasteride and tamsulosin; it is essential for the BPH station to have learned an overview of each of the major BPH trials (e.g. MTOPS, PLESS, COMBAT)

16. A

17. A

18. B

19. E

20. C

21. E

22. D

23. A

24. D

25. B

26. C

27. B

28. D

29. A – sildenafil can be prescribed with caution in peptic ulcer disease

30. E